Plant Based Diet Cookbook for Women

The Smith's Meal Plan Protocol | Quick Recipe under $3, Easy to Prepare to Reach your Ideal Weight Naturally and Kickstart your Long-Term Transformation

By Elizabeth Smith

1. Introduction

This book has been written with the express purpose to help, in a healthy and intelligent way, all

women who, for whatever reason, cannot or do not eat animal foods, and who wish to approach or

undertake a plant-based diet to keep healthy.

Studies show that using plant foods can help different categories of women.

Pregnant women: it helps to keep kidneys and blood circulation in a very good condition until

childbirth, and allows to balance moods.

Women over 50: women who have entered menopause benefit from this diet to balance

physiological functions and sometimes sudden mood swings.

Mothers with young children: eating plant-based foods allows them not to feel burdened during all

phases of the day, which we know are always chaotic

This book offers to all women, whether they are mothers, future mothers or grandmothers, varied

recipes suitable for making them discover the benefits of a plant-based diet quickly and without

stress

Enjoy the reading

Plant Based Breakfast Dishes

1) Pine Apple Smoothie

Preparation Time: 5 minutes

Cooking Time: 2 minutes

Servings: 4

Ingredients:

- 1 cup chopped pineapple (frozen or fresh)
- 1 cup chopped mango (frozen or fresh)
- ½ to 1 cup chopped kale
- ½ avocado
- ½ cup coconut milk
- 1 cup water, or coconut water
- 1 teaspoon matcha green tea powder (optional)

Directions:

1. Purée everything in a blender until smooth, adding more water (or coconut milk) if needed.

Nutrition: Calories: 566; Total fat: 36g; Carbs: 66g; Fiber: 12g; Protein: 8g

2) Choco Smoothies

Preparation Time: 5 minutes

Cooking Time: 2 minutes

Servings: 4

Ingredients:

- 1 banana
- ¼ cup rolled oats, or 1 scoop plant protein powder
- 1 tablespoon flaxseed, or chia seeds
- 1 tablespoon unsweetened cocoa powder
- 1 tablespoon peanut butter, or almond or sunflower seed butter
- 1 tablespoon maple syrup (optional)
- 1 cup alfalfa sprouts, or spinach, chopped (optional)
- ½ cup non-dairy milk (optional)
- 1 cup water

Directions:

1. Purée everything in a blender until smooth, adding more water (or non-dairy milk) if needed.
2. Add bonus boosters, as desired. Purée until blended.

Nutrition: Calories: 474; Total fat: 16g; Carbs: 79g; Fiber: 18g; Protein: 13g

3) Oats overnight

Preparation Time: 5 minutes

Cooking Time: 2 minutes

Servings: 1

Ingredients:

- ½ cup rolled oats, or quinoa flakes for gluten-free
- 1 tablespoon ground flaxseed, or chia seeds, or hemp hearts
- 1 tablespoon maple syrup, or coconut sugar (optional)
- ¼ teaspoon ground cinnamon (optional)
- TOPPING OPTIONS
- 1 apple, chopped, and 1 tablespoon walnuts
- 2 tablespoons dried cranberries and 1 tablespoon pumpkin seeds
- 1 pear, chopped, and 1 tablespoon cashews
- 1 cup sliced grapes and 1 tablespoon sunflower seeds
- 1 banana, sliced, and 1 tablespoon peanut butter
- 2 tablespoons raisins and 1 tablespoon hazelnuts
- 1 cup berries and 1 tablespoon unsweetened coconut flakes

Directions:

1. Mix the oats, flax, maple syrup, and cinnamon (if using) together in a bowl or to-go container (a travel mug or short thermos works beautifully).
2. Pour enough cool water over the oats to submerge them, and stir to combine. Leave to soak for a minimum of half an hour, or overnight.
3. Add your choice of toppings.

Nutrition: Calories: 244; Total fat: 6g; Carbs: 30g; Fiber: 6g; Protein: 7g

4) A cup of Quinoa

Preparation Time: 5 minutes

Cooking Time: 30 minutes

Servings: 2

Ingredients:

- 1 cup quinoa
- 1 teaspoon ground cinnamon
- 1 cup non-dairy milk
- 1 cup water
- 1 large banana
- 2 to 3 tablespoons unsweetened cocoa powder, or carob
- 1 to 2 tablespoons almond butter, or other nut or seed butter
- 1 tablespoon ground flaxseed, or chia or hemp seeds
- 2 tablespoons walnuts
- ¼ cup raspberries

Directions:

1. Put the quinoa, cinnamon, milk, and water in a medium pot. Bring to a boil over high heat, then turn down low and simmer, covered, for 25 to 30 minutes.

2. While the quinoa is simmering, purée or mash the banana in a medium bowl and stir in the cocoa powder, almond butter, and flaxseed.

3. To serve, spoon 1 cup cooked quinoa into a bowl, top with half the pudding and half the walnuts and raspberries.

Nutrition: Calories: 392; Total fat: 19g; Carbs: 49g; Fiber: 10g; Protein: 12g

5) Berries With Muslie

Preparation Time: 10 minutes

Cooking Time: 0 minute

Servings: 5 cups

Ingredients:

- FOR THE MUESLI
- 1 cup rolled oats
- 1 cup spelt flakes, or quinoa flakes, or more rolled oats
- 2 cups puffed cereal
- ¼ cup sunflower seeds
- ¼ cup almonds
- ¼ cup raisins
- ¼ cup dried cranberries
- ¼ cup chopped dried figs
- ¼ cup unsweetened shredded coconut
- ¼ cup non-dairy chocolate chips
- 1 to 3 teaspoons ground cinnamon
- FOR THE BOWL
- ½ cup non-dairy milk, or unsweetened applesauce
- ¾ cup muesli
- ½ cup berries

Directions:

1. Put the muesli ingredients in a container or bag and shake.

2. Combine the muesli and bowl ingredients in a bowl or to-go container.

Nutrition: Calories: 441 Total fat: 20g Carbs: 63g Fiber: 13g Protein: 10g

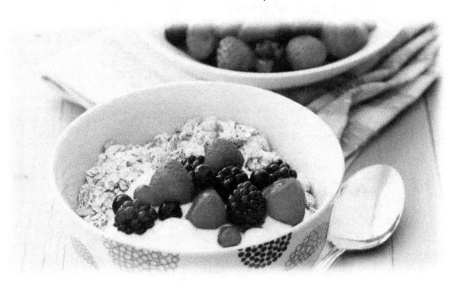

6) *Sfilatino Banana Bread*

Preparation Time: 5 minutes

Cooking Time: 1 hour + 30 minutes to cool

Servings: 1 loaf

Ingredients:

- 4 ripe bananas
- ¼ cup maple syrup
- 1 tablespoon apple cider vinegar
- 1 teaspoon vanilla extract
- 1½ cups whole-wheat flour
- ½ teaspoon ground cinnamon
- ½ teaspoon baking soda
- ¼ cup walnut pieces (optional)

Directions:

1. Preheat the oven to 350°F.
2. In a large bowl, use a fork or mixing spoon to mash the bananas until they reach a puréed consistency (small bits of banana are fine).
3. Stir in the maple syrup, apple cider vinegar, and vanilla.
4. Stir in the flour, cinnamon, and baking soda. Fold in the walnut pieces (if using).
5. Gently pour the batter into a loaf pan, filling it no more than three-quarters of the way full.
6. Bake for 1 hour, or until you can stick a knife into the middle and it comes out clean.
7. Remove from the oven and allow to cool on the countertop for a minimum of 30 minutes before serving.

Nutrition: Calories: 178; Total fat: 1g; Carbohydrates: 40g; Fiber: 5g; Protein: 4g

7) *Oatmeal Pumk*

Preparation Time: 5 minutes

Cooking Time: 35 minutes

Servings: 4

Ingredients:

- 3 cups plant-based milk
- 1 cup steel-cut oats
- 1 cup unsweetened pumpkin purée
- 2 tablespoons maple syrup
- 1 teaspoon ground cinnamon
- ⅛ teaspoon ground cloves
- ⅛ teaspoon ground nutmeg

Directions:

1. In a medium saucepan over medium-high heat, bring the milk to a boil. When a rolling boil is reached, reduce the heat to low, and stir in the oats, pumpkin purée, maple syrup, cinnamon, cloves, and nutmeg.
2. Cover and cook for 30 minutes, stirring every few minutes to ensure none of the oatmeal sticks to the bottom of the pot, and serve.

Nutrition: Calories: 218 Total fat: 5g Carbohydrates: 38g Fiber: 6g Protein: 7g

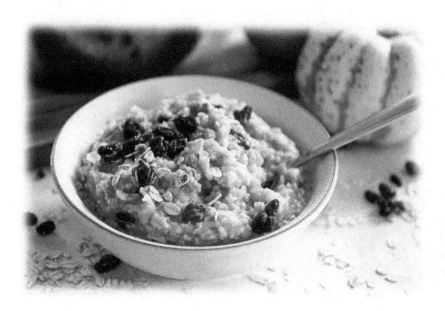

8) Burrito Veggie Breakfast

Preparation Time: 5 minutes

Cooking Time: 20 minutes

Servings: 2

Ingredients:

- ½ block (7 ounces) firm tofu
- 2 medium potatoes, cut into ¼-inch dice
- 1 cup cooked black beans, drained and rinsed
- 4 ounces' mushrooms, sliced
- 1 jalapeño, seeded and diced
- 2 tablespoons vegetable broth or water
- 1 tablespoon nutritional yeast
- ½ teaspoon garlic powder
- ½ teaspoon onion powder
- ¼ cup salsa
- 6 corn tortillas

Directions:

1. Heat a large skillet over medium-low heat.
2. Drain the tofu, then place it in the pan and mash it down with a fork or mixing spoon.
3. Stir the potatoes, black beans, mushrooms, jalapeño, broth, nutritional yeast, garlic powder, and onion powder into the skillet.
4. Reduce the heat to low, cover, and cook for 10 minutes, or until the potatoes can be easily pierced with a fork.
5. Uncover, and stir in the salsa. Cook for 5 minutes, stirring every other minute.
6. Warm the tortillas in a microwave for 15 to 30 seconds or in a warm oven until soft.
7. Remove the pan from the heat, place one-sixth of the filling in the center of each tortilla, and roll the tortillas into burritos before serving.

Nutrition: Calories: 535 Total fat: 8g Carbohydrates: 95g Fiber: 21g Protein: 29g

9) Mixed Bowl

Preparation Time: 10 minutes

Cooking Time: 30 minutes

Servings: 2

Ingredients:

- 1 ½ cups coconut milk
- 2 small-sized bananas
- 1 cup mixed berries, frozen
- 2 tablespoons almond butter
- 1 tablespoon chia seeds
- 2 tablespoons granola

Directions:

1. Add the coconut milk, bananas, berries, almond butter and chia seeds.
2. Puree until creamy, uniform and smooth.
3. Divide the blended mixture between serving bowls and top with granola. Serve immediately.

Nutrition: Calories: 533; Fat: 42.3g;Carbs: 43.4g; Protein: 6.9g

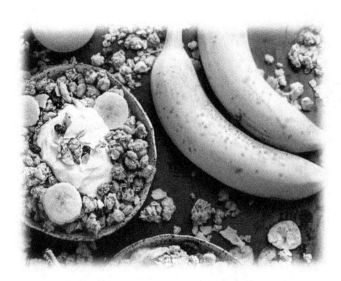

10) *Explosive Peanut Butter*

Preparation Time: 20 minutes

Cooking Time: 30 minutes

Servings: 2

Ingredients:

- 1 cup all-purpose flour
- 1/2 teaspoon baking powder
- 1/2 teaspoon sea salt
- 1 teaspoon coconut sugar
- 1/2 cup warm water
- 3 teaspoons olive oil
- 3 tablespoons peanut butter
- 3 tablespoons raspberry jam

Directions:

1. Thoroughly combine the flour, baking powder, salt and sugar.
2. Gradually add in the water until the dough comes together.
3. Divide the dough into three balls; flatten each ball to create circles.
4. Heat 1 teaspoon of the olive oil in a frying pan over a moderate flame.
5. Fry the first bread for about 9 minutes or until golden brown. Repeat with the remaining oil and dough.
6. Serve the frybread with the peanut butter and raspberry jam. Enjoy!

Nutrition: Calories: 293; Fat: 7.8g; Carbs: 50.3g; Protein: 5.5g

11) *Chia Smoothie*

Preparation Time: 20 minutes

Cooking Time: 30 minutes

Servings: 2

Ingredients:

- 1 cup coconut milk
- 2 small-sized bananas, peeled
- 1 ½ cups raspberries, fresh or frozen
- 2 dates, pitted
- 1 tablespoon coconut flakes
- 1 tablespoon pepitas
- 2 tablespoons chia seeds

Directions:

1. In your blender or food processor, mix the coconut milk with the bananas, raspberries and dates.
2. Process until creamy and smooth. Divide the smoothie between two bowls.
3. Top each smoothie bowl with the coconut flakes, pepitas and chia seeds. Bon appétit!

Nutrition: Calories: 192; Fat: 6g; Carbs: 30.5g; Protein: 5.6g

12) *Water and Beans*

Preparation Time: 20 minutes

Cooking Time: 30 minutes

Servings: 2

Ingredients:

- 2 Tbsp ground flaxseed
- 3 Tbsp water
- 2-14.5 oz cans black beans, drained and rinsed
- 1 cup panko or other breadcrumbs
- 2 tsp onion powder
- 1 tsp garlic powder
- 2 tsp cumin
- 2 tsp chili powder
- 1 tsp smoked paprika
- 1/2 tsp cayenne pepper
- 1/2 tsp kosher salt
- 1/2 tsp ground black pepper
- Oil/cooking spray, for cooking

Directions:

1. Place flax and water in a small bowl. Set aside to thicken.
2. Place beans in a large bowl and mash with potato masher or fork until you have broken up the beans.
3. Add breadcrumbs, onion powder, cumin, chili powder, garlic
4. powder, smoked paprika, cayenne pepper and salt to taste.
5. Add flax mixture and stir until all ingredients are combined.
6. Form 5 bean patties and place in the refrigerator for them to firm up.
7. Spray a large skillet with olive oil and place over medium-high heat.
8. Place patties into the large skillet and cook 10-12 minutes per side or until golden brown.
9. Serve on a bun with desired toppings.

Nutrition: Calories 439 Fat 3.1 g Carbohydrates 80.1 g Protein 24.9 g

13) *Fagotto Pull*

Preparation Time: 20 minutes

Cooking Time: 30 minutes

Servings: 2

Ingredients:

- 2 cups rolled oats. If you have a gluten sensitivity use gluten free oats.
- 1/2 cup raw pecans chopped
- 1/4 cup pumpkin seeds
- 1/4 cup almond butter
- 1/2 tsp vanilla extract
- 2 tbsp chia seeds
- 1/4 cup dried sugar-free cranberries

Directions:

1. Preheat the oven to 300°F.
2. Spray cookie sheet with non-stick spray.
3. In a large bowl, mix together oats, chopped nuts, pumpkin seeds, chia seeds, and cranberries.
4. Stir in almond butter and vanilla extract over oat mixture.
5. Combine well.
6. Pour mixture onto cookie sheet.
7. Place into the oven and bake for 9 minutes (be careful not to burn the mixture).
8. Take out of the oven and cool completely.

Nutrition: Calories 223 Fat 11.9 g Carbohydrates 25 g Protein 6.1 g

14) *Pineapple Drink*

Preparation time: 10 minutes

Cooking time: 0 minutes

Servings: 1

Ingredients:

- 1 cup coconut water
- 1 orange, peeled and cut into quarters
- 1½ cups pineapple chunks
- 1 tablespoon fresh grated ginger
- 1 teaspoon chia seeds
- 1 teaspoon turmeric powder
- A pinch of black pepper

Directions:

1. In your blender, mix the coconut water with the orange, pineapple, ginger, chia seeds, turmeric and black pepper.
2. Pulse well, pour into a glass and serve for breakfast.

Nutrition: calories 151, fat 2, fiber 6, carbs 12, protein 4

15) *Berry Peach*

Preparation Time: 5 minutes

Cooking Time: 5 minutes

Servings: 2

Ingredients:

- 1 cup of plain, unsweetened yogurt, divided
- 1 teaspoon of vanilla extract
- 1 small peach, diced
- ½ cup of blueberries

Directions:

1. Add the yogurt and vanilla in a bowl together, then add 2 tablespoons of yogurt to each of 2 cups.
2. Divide the diced peach and the blueberries between the cups, and top with the remaining yogurt.

Nutrition: Calories: 191 Total Fat: 10g Saturated Fat: 3g Cholesterol: 15mg Carbohydrates: 14g Fiber: 14g Protein: 12g Phosphorus: 189mg Potassium: 327mg Sodium: 40mg

16) *Garlic Kale Dish*

Preparation Time: 5 minutes

Cooking Time: 10 minutes

Servings: 4

Ingredients:

- 1 bunch of kale
- 2 tablespoons of oil
- 4 garlic cloves, minced

Directions:

1. Carefully tear the kale into bite-sized portions, making sure to remove the stem.
2. Discard the stems.
3. Take a large-sized pot and place it over medium heat.
4. Add oil and let it heat up.
5. Add garlic and stir for 2 minutes.
6. Add kale and cook for 5–10 minutes.
7. Serve!

Nutrition: Calories: 121 Fat: 8g Carbohydrates: 5g Protein: 4g

17) *Tofu Scramble*

Preparation Time: 5 minutes

Cooking Time: 4 minutes

Servings: 2

Ingredients:

- ½ cup of sliced white mushrooms
- ⅓ cup of medium-firm tofu, crumbled
- 1 tbsp. of chopped shallots
- ⅓ tsp. of turmeric
- 1 tsp. of cumin
- ⅓ tsp. of smoked paprika
- ½ tsp. of garlic salt
- Pepper
- 3 tbsp. of vegetable oil

Directions:

1. Heat the oil frying pan, set it on a medium, and saute the sliced mushrooms with the shallots until softened (around 3–4 minutes) over medium to high heat.
2. Add the tofu pieces and toss in the spices and the garlic salt. Toss lightly until tofu and mushrooms are nicely combined together.

Nutrition: Calories: 220 Carbohydrate: 2.59g Protein: 3.2g Sodium: 288 mg Potassium: 133.5mg Phosphorus: 68.5mg Dietary Fiber: 1.7g Fat: 23.7g

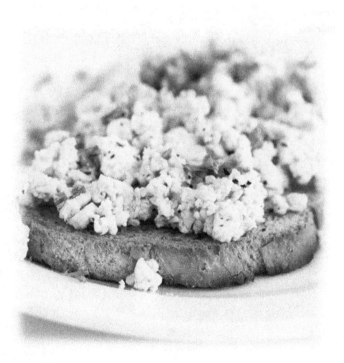

18) *Stuffed Zucchini with Carrots*

Preparation Time: 20 minutes

Cooking Time: 45 minutes

Servings: 8

Ingredients:

- 4 large zucchini
- 2 tbsp. of canola oil
- 1 diced onion
- 1 red bell pepper diced
- 1 cup of shredded carrots
- 1 summer squash diced
- 4 matzo broken into pieces
- 1 tsp. of dried oregano
- 2 tsp. of minced garlic
- 1 tsp. of ground pepper
- 1 lb. of ground chicken, cooked

Directions:

1. Preheat oven to 350°F.
2. Slice zucchini in half, lengthwise, and scoop out insides leaving ¼ inch zucchini on skins.
3. Reserve the insides.
4. Place zucchini halves skin-side down on the baking sheet.
5. In a large skillet over medium heat, warm the oil.
6. Add the onion and sauté for 3 minutes.
7. Add the zucchini insides, the rest of the veggies, the matzo, and the spices.
8. Sauté for 2 minutes.
9. Add the chicken and mix well.
10. Remove from heat and stuff the zucchini with the mixture.
11. Bake for 30 minutes.

Nutrition: Calories: 157.0 Protein: 9.5g Sodium: 49.0mg Phosphorus: 4.4mg Potassium: 236.1mg

19) *Spiced Peaches*

Preparation Time: 5 minutes

Cooking Time: 10 minutes

Servings: 2

Ingredients:

- 1 cup of canned peaches in their own juices
- 1/2 tsp. of cornstarch
- 1 tsp. of ground cloves
- 1 tsp. of ground cinnamon
- 1 tsp. of ground nutmeg
- 1/2 lemon zest
- 1/2 cup of water

Directions:

1. Drain peaches.
2. Combine water, cornstarch, cinnamon, nutmeg, ground cloves, and lemon zest in a pan on the stove.
3. Heat on medium heat and add peaches.
4. Bring to a boil, reduce the heat and simmer for 10 minutes.
5. Serve warm.

Nutrition: Calories: 70 Fat: 1g Carbohydrates: 18g Phosphorus: 26mg Potassium: 184mg Sodium: 9mg Protein: 1g

20) *Egg Fried Rice*

Preparation Time: 10 minutes

Cooking Time: 20 minutes

Servings: 6

Ingredients:

- 1 tablespoon of olive oil
- 1 tablespoon of grated peeled fresh ginger
- 1 teaspoon of minced garlic
- 1 cup of chopped carrots
- 1 scallion, white and green parts, chopped
- 2 tablespoons of chopped fresh cilantro
- 4 cups of cooked rice
- 1 tablespoon of low-sodium soy sauce
- 4 eggs, beaten

Directions:

1. In a large skillet over medium-high heat, heat the olive oil.
2. Add the ginger and garlic, and sauté until softened, about 3 minutes.
3. Add the carrots, scallion, and cilantro, and sauté until tender, about 5 minutes.
4. Stir in the rice and soy sauce, and sauté until the rice is heated through about 5 minutes.
5. Move the rice over to one side of the skillet, and pour the eggs into the empty space.
6. Scramble the eggs, then mix them into the rice.
7. Serve hot.

Nutrition: Calories: 204 Total fat: 6g Saturated fat: 1g Cholesterol: 141mg Sodium: 223mg Carbohydrates: 29g Fiber: 1g Phosphorus: 120mg Potassium: 147mg Protein: 8g

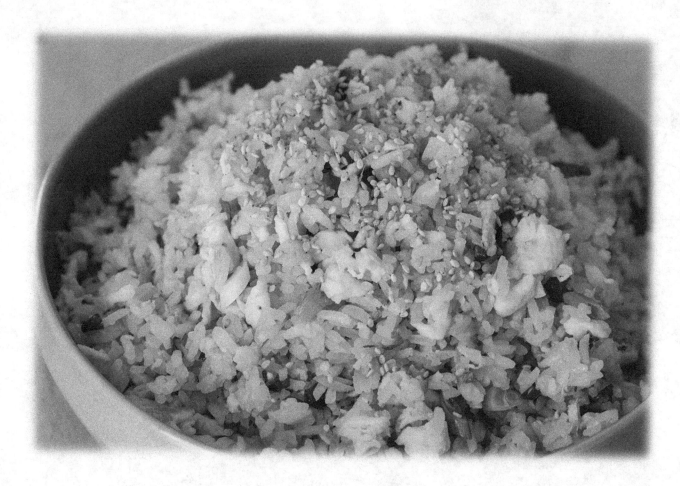

Plant Based Sides Dishes

21) Water Bath Cauliflower

Preparation Time: 5 minutes

Cooking Time: 10 minutes

Servings: 6

Ingredients:

1 large head cauliflower

1 cup water

½ teaspoon salt

1 teaspoon red pepper flakes (optional)

Directions:

1. Remove any leaves from the cauliflower, and cut it into florets.
2. In a large saucepan, bring the water to a boil.
3. Place a steamer basket over the water, and add the florets and salt. Cover and steam for 5 to 7 minutes, until tender.
4. In a large bowl, toss the cauliflower with the red pepper flakes (if using).
5. Transfer the florets to a large airtight container or 6 single-serving containers.
6. Let cool before sealing the lids.

Nutrition: Calories: 35; Fat: 0g; Protein: 3g; Carbohydrates: 7g; Fiber: 4g; Sugar: 4g; Sodium: 236mg

22) Salted Peas

Preparation Time: 5 minutes

Cooking Time: 5 minutes

Servings: 4

Ingredients:

- 1 tablespoon olive oil
- 4 cups peas, fresh or frozen (not canned)
- ½ teaspoon sea salt
- freshly ground black pepper
- 3 tablespoons chopped fresh mint

Directions:

1. In a large sauté pan, heat the olive oil over medium-high heat until hot.
2. Add the peas and cook, about 5 minutes.
3. Remove the pan from heat.
4. Stir in the salt, season with pepper, and stir in the mint.

Nutrition: Calories: 77; Fat: 3g; Protein: 4g; Carbohydrates: 12g; Fiber: 5g; Sugar: 3g;Sodium: 320mg

23) Asiasn Roasted Broccoli

Preparation Time: 5 minutes

Cooking Time: 15 minutes

Servings: 4

Ingredients:

- 1 head broccoli, cut into florets
- 2 tablespoons olive oil
- 1 tablespoon soy sauce or gluten-free tamari

Directions:

1. Preheat the oven to 425°F.
2. Line a baking sheet with parchment paper. In a large bowl, combine the broccoli, oil, and soy sauce.
3. Toss well to combine.
4. Spread the broccoli on the prepared baking sheet.
5. Roast for 10 minutes.
6. Toss the broccoli with a spatula and roast for an additional 5 minutes, or until the edges of the florets begin to brown.

Nutrition: Calories: 44; Fat: 2g; Protein: 3g; Carbohydrates: 7g; Fiber: 2g; Sugar: 3g; Sodium: 20mg

24) *Linguine Shaded with Wine*

Preparation time: 10 minutes

Cooking time: 18 minutes

Servings: 4

Ingredients:

- 1 tablespoon olive oil
- 5 garlic cloves, minced
- 16 oz shiitake, chopped
- ¼ teaspoon salt
- ¼ teaspoon ground pepper
- 1 pinch red pepper flakes
- ½ cup dry white wine
- 12 oz linguine
- 2 teaspoons vegan butter
- ¼ cup Italian parsley, finely chopped

Directions:

1. Fill a suitably-sized pot with salted water and bring it to a boil on high heat.
2. Add pasta to the boiling water then cook until it is al dente, then rinse under cold water.
3. Place a non-stick skillet over medium-high heat then add olive oil.
4. Stir in garlic and sauté for 1 minute.
5. Stir in mushrooms and cook for 10 minutes.
6. Add salt, red pepper flakes, and black pepper for seasoning.
7. Toss in the cooked pasta and mix well.
8. Garnish with parsley and butter.

Nutrition: Calories: 40; Fat: 2.0g; Protein: 5g; Carbohydrates: 7g; Fiber: 4g; Sugar: 3g; Sodium: 18mg

25) *Plant Based Low Carb*

Preparation Time: 20 minutes

Cooking Time: 30 minutes

Servings: 2

Ingredients:

- 2 tablespoons carrots, shredded
- 1 package kelp noodles, soaked in water
- 1 cup broccoli, frozen
- For the Sauce
- 1 tablespoon sesame oil
- 2 tablespoons tamari
- ½ teaspoon ground ginger
- ¼ teaspoon Sriracha
- ½ teaspoon garlic powder

Directions:

1. Put the broccoli in a saucepan on medium low heat and add the sauce ingredients.
2. Cook for about 5 minutes and add the noodles after draining water.
3. Allow to simmer about 10 minutes, occasionally stirring to avoid burning.
4. When the noodles have softened, mix everything well and dish out to serve.

Nutrition: Calories: 30; Fat: 3.5.0g; Protein: 6g; Carbohydrates: 6g; Fiber: 4g;

26) *Veggie Chow*

Preparation Time: 20 minutes

Cooking Time: 30 minutes

Servings: 2

Ingredients:

- ½ large onion, chopped
- ½ small leek, chopped
- ½ tablespoon ginger paste
- ½ tablespoon Worcester sauce
- ½ tablespoon Oriental seasoning
- ½ teaspoon parsley
- Salt and black pepper, to taste
- ½ pound noodles
- 2 large carrots, diced
- 2 celery sticks, chopped
- 1 tablespoon olive oil
- ½ teaspoon garlic paste
- 1½ tablespoons soy sauce
- 1 tablespoon Chinese five spice
- ½ teaspoon coriander
- 2 cups water

Directions:

1. Put olive oil, ginger, garlic paste, and onion in a pot on medium heat and sauté for about 5 minutes.
2. Stir in all the vegetables and cook for about5 minutes.
3. Add rest of the ingredients and combine well.
4. Secure the lid and cook on medium heat for about 20 minutes, stirring occasionally.
5. Open the lid and dish out to serve hot.

Nutrition: Calories: 30; Fat: 3.5.0g; Protein: 6g; Carbohydrates: 6g; Fiber: 4g;Sugar: 5g; Sodium: 18mg

27) 5 min Veggie pasta

Preparation Time: 5 minutes

Cooking Time: 16 minutes

Servings: 4

Ingredients:

- 3 shallots, chopped
- ¼ teaspoon red pepper flakes
- ¼ cup vegan parmesan cheese
- 2 tablespoons olive oil
- 2 garlic cloves, minced
- 8-ounces spinach leaves
- 8-ounces linguine pasta
- 1 pinch salt
- 1 pinch black pepper

Directions:

1. Boil salted water in a large pot and add pasta.
2. Cook for about 6 minutes and drain the pasta in a colander.
3. Heat olive oil over medium heat in a large skillet and add the shallots.
4. Cook for about 5 minutes until soft and caramelized and stir in the spinach, garlic, red pepper flakes, salt and black pepper.
5. Cook for about 5 minutes and add pasta and 2 ladles of pasta water.
6. Stir in the parmesan cheese and dish out in a bowl to serve.

Nutrition: Calories: 25; Fat: 2.0g; Protein: 5.2g; Carbohydrates: 5.3g; Fiber: 4g; Sodium: 18mg

28) Sweet Potatoes with Black Bean

Preparation Time: 5 minutes

Cooking Time: 1 hour

Servings: 4

Ingredients:

- 4 sweet potatoes
- 15 oz. cooked black beans
- ½ tsp. ground black pepper
- ½ red onion, peeled, diced
- ½ tsp. sea salt
- ¼ tsp. onion powder
- ¼ tsp. garlic powder
- ¼ tsp. red chili powder
- ¼ tsp. cumin
- 1 tsp. lime juice
- 1 ½ tbsps. olive oil
- ½ c. cashew cream sauce

Directions:

1. Spread sweet potatoes on a baking tray greased with oil and bake for 65 minutes at 350 degrees' f until tender.
2. Meanwhile, prepare the sauce, and for this, whisk together the cream sauce, black pepper, and lime juice until combined, set aside until required.
3. When 10 minutes of the baking time of potatoes are left, heat a skillet pan with oil. Add in onion to cook until golden for 5 minutes.
4. Then stir in spice, cook for another 3 minutes, stir in bean until combined and cook for 5 minutes until hot.
5. Let roasted sweet potatoes cool for 10 minutes, then cut them open, mash the flesh and top with bean mixture, cilantro and avocado, and then drizzle with cream sauce.
6. Serve straight away.

Nutrition: Calories: 387, Fat: 16.1 g, Carbs: 53 g, Protein: 10.4 g

29) Chickpea with Cocco

Preparation Time: 5 minutes

Cooking Time: 15 minutes

Servings: 4

Nutrition: Calories: 225, Fat: 9.4 g, Carbs: 28.5 g, Protein: 7.3 g

Ingredients:

- 2 tsps. coconut flour
- 16 oz. cooked chickpeas
- 14 oz. tomatoes, diced
- 1 red onion, sliced
- 1 ½ tsps. minced garlic
- ½ tsp. sea salt
- 1 tsp. curry powder
- 1/3 tsp. ground black pepper
- 1 ½ tbsps. garam masala
- ¼ tsp. cumin
- 1 lime, juiced
- oz. coconut milk, unsweetened
- 2 tbsps. coconut oil

Directions:

1. Take a large pot, place it over medium-high heat, add oil and when it melts, add onions and tomatoes, season with salt and black pepper and cook for 5 minutes.
2. Switch heat to medium-low level, cook for 10 minutes until tomatoes have released their liquid, then add chickpeas and stir in garlic, curry powder, garam masala, and cumin until combined.
3. Stir in milk and flour, bring the mixture to boil, then switch heat to medium heat and simmer the curry for 12 minutes until cooked.
4. Taste to adjust seasoning, drizzle with lime juice, and serve.

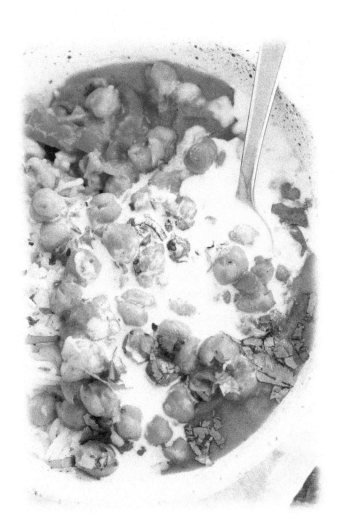

30) *Pilaf with Garbanzos Apricots*

Preparation Time: 5 minutes

Cooking Time: 20 minutes

Servings: 4

Ingredients:

- 1 c. bulgur
- 6 oz. cooked chickpeas
- ½ c. dried apricot
- 1 white onion, peeled, diced
- ½ tsps. minced garlic
- 2 tsps. curry powder
- ½ tsp. salt
- 1 tbsp. olive oil
- ¼ c. fresh parsley leaves
- 2 c. vegetable broth
- ¾ c. water

Nutrition: Calories: 222, Fat: 4.5 g, Carbs: 35 g, Protein: 9.5 g

Directions:

1. Take a saucepan, place it over high heat, pour in water and 1 ½ cup broth, and bring it to a boil.
2. Then stir in bulgur, switch heat to medium-low level and simmer for 15 minutes until most of the liquid has absorbed.
3. Meanwhile, take a skillet pan, place it over medium heat, add oil and when hot, add onion, cook for 10 minutes, then stir in garlic and curry powder and cook for another minute.
4. Then add apricots, beans, and salt, pour in remaining broth and bring the mixture to boiling.
5. Remove pan from heat, fluff the bulgur with a fork, add to the onion-apricot mixture and stir until mixed.
6. Garnish with parsley and serve.

31) *Eggplant Soup*

Preparation Time: 20 minutes

Cooking Time: 40 minutes

Servings: 6

Ingredients:

- Sweet onion – 1 small, cut into quarters
- Small red bell peppers – 2, halved
- Cubed eggplant – 2 cups
- Garlic – 2 cloves, crushed
- Olive oil – 1 Tbsp.
- Chicken stock – 1 cup
- Water
- Chopped fresh basil – ¼ cup
- Ground black pepper

Nutrition: Calories: 61 Fat: 2g Carb: 9g Phosphorus: 33mg Potassium: 198mg Sodium: 98mg Protein: 2g

Directions:

1. Preheat the oven to 350F.
2. Put the onions, red peppers, eggplant, and garlic in a baking dish.
3. Drizzle the vegetables with the olive oil.
4. Roast the vegetables for 30 minutes or until they are slightly charred and soft.
5. Cool the vegetables slightly and remove the skin from the peppers.
6. Puree the vegetables with a hand mixer (with the chicken stock).
7. Transfer the soup to a medium pot and add enough water to reach the desired thickness.
8. Heat the soup to a simmer and add the basil.
9. Season with pepper and serve.

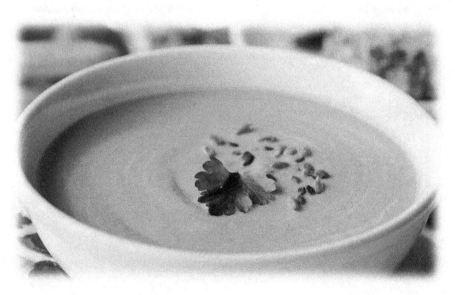

32) *Kale Chips*

Preparation Time: 20 minutes

Cooking Time: 25 minutes

Servings: 6

Ingredients:

- Kale – 2 cups
- Olive oil – 2 tsp.
- Chili powder – ¼ tsp.
- Pinch cayenne pepper

Nutrition: Calories: 24 Fat: 2g Carb: 2g Phosphorus: 21mg Potassium: 111mg Sodium: 13mg Protein: 1g

Directions:

1. Preheat the oven to 300F.
2. Line 2 baking sheets with parchment paper; set aside.
3. Remove the stems from the kale and tear the leaves into 2-inch pieces.
4. Wash the kale and dry it completely.
5. Transfer the kale to a large bowl and drizzle with olive oil.
6. Use your hands to toss the kale with oil, taking care to coat each leaf evenly.
7. Season the kale with chili powder and cayenne pepper and toss to combine thoroughly.
8. Spread the seasoned kale in a single layer on each baking sheet. Do not overlap the leaves.
9. Bake the kale, rotating the pans once, for 20 to 25 minutes until it is crisp and dry.
10. Remove the trays from the oven and allow the chips to cool on the trays for 5 minutes.
11. Serve.

33) *Omelette Penne*

Preparation Time: 15 minutes

Cooking Time: 30 minutes

Servings: 4

Ingredients:

- Egg whites- 6
- Rice milk – ¼ cup
- Chopped fresh parsley – 1 Tbsp.
- Chopped fresh thyme – 1 tsp.
- Chopped fresh chives – 1 tsp.
- Ground black pepper
- Olive oil – 2 tsps.
- Small sweet onion – ¼, chopped
- Minced garlic – 1 tsp.
- Boiled and chopped red bell pepper – ½ cup
- Cooked penne – 2 cups

Nutrition: Calories: 170 Fat: 3g Carb: 25g Phosphorus: 62mg Potassium: 144mg Sodium: 90mg Protein: 10g

Directions:

1. Preheat the oven to 350F.
2. In a bowl, whisk together the egg whites, rice milk, parsley, thyme, chives, and pepper.
3. Heat the oil in a skillet.
4. Sauté the onion, garlic, red pepper for 4 minutes or until they are softened.
5. Add the cooked penne to the skillet.
6. Pour the egg mixture over the pasta and shake the pan to coat the pasta.
7. Leave the skillet on the heat for 1 minute to set the bottom of the frittata and then transfer the skillet to the oven.
8. Bake, the frittata for 25 minutes or until it is set and golden brown.
9. Serve.

34) Cauliflower Balls

Preparation Time: 5 minutes

Cooking Time: 8 minutes

Servings: 4

Nutrition: Calories: 227 Fat: 12g Carb: 15g Phosphorus: 193mg Potassium: 513mg Sodium: 158mg Protein: 13g.

Ingredients:

- Eggs – 2
- Egg whites – 2
- Onion – ½, diced
- Cauliflower – 2 cups, frozen
- All-purpose white flour – 2 Tbsps.
- Black pepper – 1 tsp.
- Coconut oil – 1 Tbsp.
- Curry powder – 1 tsp.
- Fresh cilantro – 1 Tbsp

Directions:

1. Soak vegetables in warm water prior to cooking.
2. Steam cauliflower over a pan of boiling water for 10 minutes.
3. Blend eggs and onion in a food processor before adding cooked cauliflower, spices, cilantro, flour, and pepper and blast in the processor for 30 seconds.
4. Heat a skillet on a high heat and add oil.
5. Pour tbsp. portions of the cauliflower mixture into the pan and brown on each side until crispy, about 3 to 4 minutes.
6. Enjoy with a salad.

35) Tomatoes Mix ans Basil

Preparation Time: 10 minutes

Cooking Time: 14 minutes

Servings: 2

Ingredients:

- 1 bunch basil, chopped
- 3 garlic clove, minced
- A drizzle of olive oil
- Salt and black pepper to the taste
- 2 cups cherry tomatoes, halved

Directions:

1. In a pan that fits your Air Fryer, combine tomatoes with garlic, salt, pepper, basil and oil, toss, introduce in your Air Fryer and cook at 320 ° F for 12 minutes.
2. Divide between plates and serve as a side dish.

Nutrition: Calories 242 Total Fat 7.6 g Saturated 2.6 g Cholesterol 0 mg Sodium 115 mg Total Carbs 29.1 g Fiber 4.6 g Sugar 6 g Protein 14.2 g

36) Gold Potatoes and Bell Pepper Mix

Preparation Time: 10 minutes

Cooking Time: 25 minutes

Servings: 3

Ingredients:

- 4 gold potatoes, cubed
- 1 yellow onion, chopped
- 2 teaspoons olive oil
- 1 green bell pepper, chopped
- Salt and black pepper to the taste
- ½ teaspoon thyme, dried

Directions:

1. Heat up your Air Fryer at 350 ° F, add oil, heat it up, add onion, bell pepper, salt and pepper, stir and cook for 5 minutes.
2. Add potatoes and thyme, stir, cover and cook at 360 °F for 20 minutes.
3. Divide between plates and serve as a side dish.

Nutrition: Calories 242 Total Fat 7.6 g Saturated 2.6 g Cholesterol 0 mg Sodium 115 mg Total Carbs 29.1 g Fiber 4.6 g Sugar 6 g Protein 14.2 g

37) *Pamplona rice*

Preparation time: 3 hours and 10 minutes

Cooking time: 40 minutes

Servings: 10

Nutrition: Calories 242 Total Fat 7.6 g Saturated 2.6 g Cholesterol 0 mg Sodium 115 mg Total Carbs 29.1 g Fiber 4.6 g Sugar 6 g Protein 14.2 g

Ingredients:

- 1 cup of long grain rice, uncooked
- 1/2 cup of chopped green bell pepper
- 14 ounce of diced tomatoes
- 1/2 cup of chopped white onion
- 1 teaspoon of minced garlic
- 1/2 teaspoon of salt
- 1 teaspoon of red chili powder
- 1 teaspoon of ground cumin
- 4-ounce of tomato puree
- 8 fluid ounce of water

Directions:

1. Grease a 6-quarts slow cooker with a non-stick cooking spray and add all the ingredients into it.
2. Stir properly and cover the top.
3. Plug in the slow cooker; adjust the cooking time to 5 hours and let it cook on the high heat setting or until the rice absorbs all the liquid.
4. Serve right away.

38) *Super Veggie Chili*

Preparation time: 2 hours and 10 minutes

Cooking time: 5 minutes

Servings: 6

Ingredients:

- 16-ounce of vegetarian baked beans
- 16 ounce of cooked chickpeas
- 16 ounce of cooked kidney beans
- 15 ounce of cooked corn
- 1 medium-sized green bell pepper, cored and chopped
- 2 stalks of celery, peeled and chopped
- 12 ounce of chopped tomatoes
- 1 medium-sized white onion, peeled and chopped
- 1 teaspoon of minced garlic
- 1 teaspoon of salt
- 1 tablespoon of red chili powder
- 1 tablespoon of dried oregano
- 1 tablespoon of dried basil
- 1 tablespoon of dried parsley
- 18-ounce of black bean soup
- 4-ounce of tomato puree

Directions:

1. Take a 6-quarts slow cooker, grease it with a non-stick cooking spray and place all the ingredients into it.
2. Stir properly and cover the top.
3. Plug in the slow cooker; adjust the cooking time to 2 hours and let it cook on the high heat setting or until it is cooked thoroughly.
4. Serve right away.

Nutrition: Calories 242 Total Fat 7.6 g Saturated 2.6 g Cholesterol 0 mg Sodium 115 mg Total Carbs 29.1 g Fiber 4.6 g Sugar 6 g Protein 14.2 g

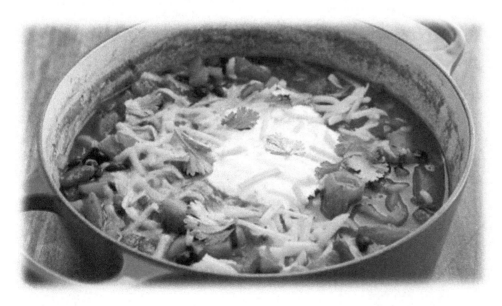

39) Sweet Potato & Curry

Preparation time: 6 hours and 20 minutes

Cooking time: 5 minutes

Servings: 6

Nutrition: Calories 242 Total Fat 7.6 g Saturated 2.6 g Cholesterol 0 mg Sodium 115 mg Total Carbs 29.1 g Fiber 4.6 g Sugar 6 g Protein 14.2 g

Ingredients:

- 2 pounds of sweet potatoes, peeled and chopped
- 1/2 pound of red cabbage, shredded
- 2 red chilies, seeded and sliced
- 2 medium-sized red bell peppers, cored and sliced
- 2 large white onions, peeled and sliced
- 1 1/2 teaspoon of minced garlic
- 1 teaspoon of grated ginger
- 1/2 teaspoon of salt
- 1 teaspoon of paprika
- 1/2 teaspoon of cayenne pepper
- 2 tablespoons of peanut butter
- 4 tablespoons of olive oil
- 12-ounce of tomato puree
- 14 fluid ounce of coconut milk
- 1/2 cup of chopped coriander

Directions:

1. Place a large non-stick skillet pan over an average heat, add 1 tablespoon of oil and let it heat. Then add the onion and cook for 10 minutes or until it gets soft.
2. Add the garlic, ginger, salt, paprika, cayenne pepper and continue cooking for 2 minutes or until it starts producing fragrance. Transfer this mixture to a 6-quarts slow cooker, and reserve the pan.
3. In the pan, add 1 tablespoon of oil and let it heat.
4. Add the cabbage, red chili, bell pepper and cook it for 5 minutes.
5. Then transfer this mixture to the slow cooker and reserve the pan.
6. Add the remaining oil to the pan; the sweet potatoes in a single layer and cook it in 3 batches for 5 minutes or until it starts getting brown. Add the sweet potatoes to the slow cooker, along with tomato puree, coconut milk and stir properly.
7. Cover the top, plug in the slow cooker; adjust the cooking time to 6 hours and let it cook on the low heat setting or until the sweet potatoes are tender.
8. When done, add the seasoning and pour it in the peanut butter.
9. Garnish it with coriander and serve.

40) Chicpea Wraps

Preparation time: 15 minutes

Cooking time: 0 minutes

Servings: 3

Ingredients:

- 3 tablespoons tahini
- 1 tablespoon curry powder
- ¼ teaspoon sea salt (optional)
- Zest and juice of 1 lime
- 3 to 4 tablespoons water
- 1½ cups cooked chickpeas
- 1 cup diced mango
- ½ cup fresh cilantro, chopped
- 1 red bell pepper, deseeded and diced
- 3 large whole-wheat wraps
- 1½ cups shredded lettuce

Directions:

1. In a large bowl, stir together the tahini, curry powder, lime zest, lime juice and sea salt (if desired) until smooth and creamy. Whisk in 3 to 4 tablespoons water to help thin the mixture.
2. Add the cooked chickpeas, mango, cilantro and bell pepper to the bowl. Toss until well coated.
3. On a clean work surface, lay the wraps. Divide the chickpea and mango mixture among the wraps. Spread the shredded lettuce on top and roll up tightly.
4. Serve immediately.

Nutrition: calories: 436fat: 17.9g carbs: 8.9g protein: 15.2g fiber: 12.1g

Plant Based Vegetables Dishes

41) Veggie Falafel

Preparation Time: 20 minutes

Cooking Time: 30 minutes

Servings: 8

Nutrition: Protein: 16% 19 kcal Fat: 24% 29 kcal Carbohydrates: 60% 71 kcal

Ingredients:

- 1 tbsp. extra-virgin olive oil
- 1 cup dried chickpeas soaked for 24 hours in the refrigerator
- 1 cup cauliflower, chopped
- ½ cup red onion, chopped
- ½ cup packed fresh parsley
- 2 cloves garlic, quartered
- 1 tsp. sea salt
- ½ tsp. ground black pepper
- ½ tsp. ground cumin
- ¼ tsp. ground cinnamon

Directions:

1. Preheat oven to 375° F.
2. In a food processor, mix chickpeas, cauliflower, onion, parsley, garlic, salt, pepper, cumin seeds, cinnamon, and olive oil until mixture is smooth.
3. Take 2 tbsps. of mixture and make the falafel into small patties.
4. Keep falafel on greased baking tray.
5. Bake falafel for about 25 to 30 minutes in preheated oven until golden brown from both sides.
6. Once cooked remove from oven.

42) Blueberries Ice Cream

Preparation Time: 5 minutes

Cooking Time: 0 minute

Servings: 4

Nutrition: Protein: 3% 4 kcal Fat: 40% 60 kcal Carbohydrates: 57% 86 kcal

Ingredients:

- 1/4 Cup Coconut Cream
- 1 Tbsp. Maple Syrup
- ¼ Cup Coconut Flour
- 1 Cup Blueberries
- ¼ Cup Blueberries for Topping

Directions:

1. Put ingredients into food processor and mix well on high speed.
2. Pour mixture in silicon molds and freeze in freezer for about 2-4 hours.
3. Once balls are set remove from freezer.
4. Top with berries.

43) Healty Chocolate Puddin

Preparation Time: 5 minutes

Cooking Time: 0 minute

Servings: 2

Nutrition: Protein: 3% 7 kcal Fat: 83% 163 kcal Carbohydrates: 13% 26 kcal

Ingredients:

- 1/2 Cup Coconut Milk
- 1 Tsp. Maple Syrup
- 1-3 Tbsps. Cocoa Powder
- Pinch Instant Coffee
- 2 Tbsps. Coconut Cream
- Blackberries for Topping

Directions:

1. Heat up coconut milk and maple syrup until it just begins to simmer.
2. Add cocoa and coffee in milk mixture.
3. Add cream to same mixture and whip until relatively stiff peaks form.
4. Transfer to a serving glass.
5. Chill the mousse in freezer for 2-3 hours.
6. Top with some berries and spoon of coconut cream.

44) Chocolate Turron

Preparation Time: 10 minutes

Cooking Time: 5 minutes

Servings: 16

Nutrition: 120 calories, 2g proteins, 10g fats, 10g carbs

Ingredients:

- ½ lb dark chopped chocolate
- 2 tablespoons melted coconut oil
- 2 ounces unsalted raw hazelnuts

Directions:

1. Place dark chocolate in a saucepan. Cook over medium heat, stirring occasionally until chocolate is melted.
2. Remove chocolate from the heat. Add hazelnuts, and combine well.
3. Pour the chocolate-hazelnuts mixture into lined rectangular dish.
4. Cool to room temperature. Chop the turron.
5. If it's too hot in the room, keep turron in the fridge.

45) Coconut Balls

Preparation Time: 20 minutes, 1 week for freezing

Cooking Time: 0 minute

Servings: 1

Ingredients:

- 3 ounces shredded coconut
- 1-ounce almond flour
- 3 ounces' agave syrup

Nutrition: 88 calories, 1g proteins, 5g fats, 9g carbs

Directions:

1. Mix shredded coconut, flour, and syrup in a food processor until well combined.
2. Make 10 balls using your hands.
3. Roll the balls in 1 oz shredded coconut.
4. You can keep these balls in a sealed container in a fridge for one week.

46) Potato and Carrots Salad

Preparation Time: 15 minutes

Cooking Time: 10 minutes

Servings: 6

Nutrition: Calories 106 Fat 5.3 g Saturated fat 1 g Carbohydrates 12.6 g Fiber 1.8g Protein 2 g

Ingredients:

- Water
- 6 potatoes, sliced into cubes
- 3 carrots, sliced into cubes
- 1 tablespoon milk
- 1 tablespoon Dijon mustard
- ¼ cup mayonnaise
- Pepper to taste
- 2 teaspoons fresh thyme, chopped
- 1 stalk celery, chopped
- 2 scallions, chopped
- 1 slice turkey bacon, cooked crispy and crumbled

Directions:

1. Fill your pot with water.
2. Place it over medium high heat.
3. Boil the potatoes and carrots for 10 minutes or until tender.
4. Drain and let cool.
5. In a bowl, mix the milk mustard, mayo, pepper and thyme.
6. Stir in the potatoes, carrots and celery.
7. Coat evenly with the sauce.
8. Cover and refrigerate for 4 hours.
9. Top with the scallions and turkey bacon bits before serving.

47) Snap Pea Salad

Preparation Time: 1 hour

Cooking Time: 0 minute

Servings: 6

Nutrition: Calories 69 Fat 3.7 g Saturated fat 0.6 g Carbohydrates 7.1 g Fiber 1.8 g Protein 2 g

Ingredients:

- 2 tablespoons mayonnaise
- ¾ teaspoon celery seed
- ¼ cup cider vinegar
- 1 teaspoon yellow mustard
- 1 tablespoon sugar
- Salt and pepper to taste
- 4 oz. radishes, sliced thinly
- 12 oz. sugar snap peas, sliced thinly

Directions:

1. In a bowl, combine the mayonnaise, celery seeds, vinegar, mustard, sugar, salt and pepper.
2. Stir in the radishes and snap peas.
3. Refrigerate for 30 minutes.

48) Avocado Salad

Preparation Time: 10 minutes

Cooking Time: 0 minute

Servings: 4

Nutrition: Calories 224 Fat 18 g Saturated fat 3.9 g Carbohydrates 6.1 g Fiber 3.6 g Protein 10.6 g

Ingredients:

- 1 avocado
- 6 hard-boiled eggs, peeled and chopped
- 1 tablespoon mayonnaise
- 2 tablespoons freshly squeezed lemon juice
- ¼ cup celery, chopped
- 2 tablespoons chives, chopped
- Salt and pepper to taste

Directions:

1. Add the avocado to a large bowl.
2. Mash the avocado using a fork.
3. Stir in the egg and mash the eggs.
4. Add the mayo, lemon juice, celery, chives, salt and pepper.
5. Chill in the refrigerator for at least 30 minutes before serving.

49) Pepper Salad

Preparation Time: 1 hour and 25 minutes

Cooking Time: 0 minute

Servings: 8

Nutrition: Calories 116 Fat 7 g Saturated fat 2 g Carbohydrates 11 g Fiber 2 g Protein 3 g

Ingredients:

- 2 tablespoons balsamic vinegar
- 2 tablespoons olive oil
- ½ teaspoon Dijon mustard
- 2 teaspoons fresh basil leaves, chopped
- 1 tablespoon fresh chives, chopped
- 1 teaspoon sugar
- Pepper to taste
- 2 cups yellow bell peppers, sliced into rings
- 1 cups orange bell pepper, sliced into rings
- 4 tomatoes, sliced into rounds
- ¼ cup blue cheese, crumbled

Directions:

1. Mix the vinegar, olive oil, mustard, basil, chives, sugar and pepper in a bowl.
2. Arrange the tomatoes and pepper rings in a serving plate.
3. Sprinkle the crumbled blue cheese on top.
4. Drizzle with the dressing.
5. Chill in the refrigerator for 1 hour before serving.

50) Arugula Radicchio Salad

Preparation Time: 15 minutes

Cooking Time: 0 minute

Servings: 4

Nutrition: Calories 85 Fat 6.6 g Saturated fat 0.5 g Carbohydrates 5.1 g Fiber 1 g Protein 2.2 g

Ingredients:

- 6 cups fresh arugula leaves
- 2 cups radicchio, chopped
- ¼ cup low-fat balsamic vinaigrette
- ¼ cup pine nuts, toasted and chopped

Directions:

1. Arrange the arugula leaves in a serving bowl.
2. Sprinkle the radicchio on top.
3. Drizzle with the vinaigrette.
4. Sprinkle the pine nuts on top.

51) Tuna Salad

Preparation Time: 4 hours and 20 minutes

Cooking Time: 10 minutes

Servings: 6

Nutrition: Calories 243 Fat 9.9 g Saturated fat 2 g Carbohydrates 22.2 g Fiber 4.6 g Protein 17.5 g

Ingredients:

- Water
- 3 potatoes, peeled and sliced into cubes
- ½ cup plain yogurt
- ½ cup mayonnaise
- 1 clove garlic, crushed and minced
- 1 tablespoon almond milk
- 1 tablespoon fresh dill, chopped
- ½ teaspoon lemon zest
- Salt to taste
- 1 cup cucumber, chopped
- ¼ cup scallions, chopped
- ¼ cup radishes, chopped
- 9 oz. canned tuna flakes
- 2 hard-boiled eggs, chopped
- 6 cups lettuce, chopped

Directions:

1. Fill your pot with water.
2. Add the potatoes and boil.
3. Cook for 10 minutes or until slightly tender.
4. Drain and let cool.
5. In a bowl, mix the yogurt, mayo, garlic, almond milk, fresh dill, lemon zest and salt.
6. Stir in the potatoes, tuna flakes and eggs.
7. Mix well.
8. Chill in the refrigerator for 4 hours.
9. Stir in the shredded lettuce before serving.

52) High Protein Salad

Preparation Time: 5 minutes

Cooking Time: 5 minutes

Servings: 4

Nutrition: Calories: 205 Fat: 2 g Protein: 13 g Carbs: 31 g Fiber: 17g

Ingredients:

- 1 15-oz can green kidney beans
- 2 4 tbsp capers
- 3 4 handfuls arugula
- 4 15-oz can lentils
- 5 1 tbsp caper brine
- 6 1 tbsp tamari
- 7 1 tbsp balsamic vinegar
- 8 2 tbsp peanut butter
- 9 2 tbsp hot sauce
- 10 1 tbsp tahini

Directions:

For the dressing:

1. In a bowl, whisk together all the ingredients until they come together to form a smooth dressing.

For the salad:

2. Mix the beans, arugula, capers, and lentils. Top with the dressing and serve.

53) Veggie Rice Bowl

Preparation Time: 5 minutes

Cooking Time: 15 minutes

Servings: 6

Nutrition: Calories: 260 Fat: 9 g Protein: 9 g Carbs: 36 g Fiber: 5g

Ingredients:

- 2 tbsp coconut oil
- 1 tsp ground cumin
- 1 tsp ground turmeric
- 1 tsp chili powder
- 1 red bell pepper, chopped
- 1 tsp tomato paste
- 1 bunch of broccoli, cut into bite-sized florets with short stems
- 1 tsp salt, to taste
- 1 large red onion, sliced
- 2 garlic cloves, minced
- 1 head of cauliflower, cut into bite-sized florets
- 2 cups cooked rice (or other cooked grain)
- Freshly ground black pepper to taste

Directions:

1. In a large pan or skillet, heat the coconut oil over medium-high heat. When the oil is hot, stir in the turmeric, cumin, chili powder, salt, and tomato paste.

2. Cook the content for 1 minute. Stir repeatedly until the spices are fragrant. Add the garlic and onion. Sauté for 2 to 3 minutes until the onions are softened.

3. Add the broccoli, cauliflower, and bell pepper. Cover. Cook for 3 to 4 minutes and stir occasionally. Add the cooked rice. Stir so it will combine well with the vegetables. Cook for 2 to 3 minutes. Stir until the rice is warmed through. Check the seasoning and adjust to taste if desired.

4. Lower the heat and cook on low for 2 to 3 more minutes so the flavors will meld.

5. Serve with freshly ground black pepper.

54) Red Beans in a Bowl

Preparation Time: 5 minutes

Cooking Time: 25 minutes

Servings: 4

Nutrition: Calories: 221 Fat: 1 g Protein: 11 g Carbs: 25 g Fiber: 4g

Ingredients:

- 3½ cups water, divided
- 1 tsp red pepper flakes
- 3 stalks celery, diced
- 1 green pepper, chopped
- ½ yellow onion, diced
- 2 small cans kidney beans, drained and rinsed
- 1 cup brown rice
- 3 garlic cloves, minced
- 1 bay leaf
- 1 tsp sage
- ½ tsp oregano
- ½ tsp cayenne

Directions:

1. Add 1 cup of rice and 2 cups of water to a pot.

2. Bring the contents to a boil, turn down the heat, and cover to simmer until the water is absorbed.

3. Once the rice is cooked, on low-medium heat, put all the remaining ingredients in a large saucepan and cover for 20 to 30 minutes.

4. Stir occasionally until the onions are cooked and the 1 cup of water has boiled off.

5. Serve and enjoy.

55) Grilled Asparagus with Cheakpea

Preparation Time: 5 minutes

Cooking Time: 8 minutes

Servings: 2

Nutrition: Calories: 270 Fat: 3 g Protein: 14 g Carbs: 52 g

Ingredients:

- 2 slices sourdough bread
- 10 Asparagus spears
- 4 tbsp chickpea flour
- 2 tbsp nutritional yeast (optional)
- 1 tsp black salt (optional)
- ½ tsp garlic powder
- Pepper and salt, to taste

Directions:

1. Preheat the grill. Mix the nutritional yeast, chickpea flour, garlic powder, and black salt (if you are using).
2. Stir in 1 tbsp of water until you get a thick and pourable consistency.
3. Spread the mixture on the bread slices. Arrange the asparagus spears on top.
4. Grill for about 8 minutes until the chickpea mixture firms up and the asparagus is properly cooked.
5. Serve on its own or with mushrooms or grilled tomatoes.
6. Enjoy!

56) Pickled Garlic Okra

Preparation Time: 5 minutes

Cooking Time: 10 minutes

Servings: 40

Nutrition: Calories 28 Fat 1.7 g Saturated fat 0 g Carbohydrates 3.2 g Fiber 0.7 g Protein 0.4 g Cholesterol 0 mg Sugars 1 g Sodium 165 mg Potassium 65 mg

Ingredients:

- 2 lb. okra
- 2 cups black olives, pitted and rinsed
- 8 cloves garlic, crushed and minced
- 2 teaspoons fennel seed
- 32 basil leaves, chopped
- 6 cups rice vinegar
- 2 cups water
- 4 teaspoons salt
- ¼ cup sugar

Directions:

1. Add the okra, black olives, garlic, fennel seeds and basil leaves in glass jars with lids.
2. In a pan over medium high heat, boil the vinegar, water, salt and sugar.
3. Reduce heat and simmer for 5 minutes.
4. Let cool.
5. Add the mixture to the glass jars.
6. Refrigerate for 24 hours.

57) Stuffed Cauliflower

Preparation Time: 5 minutes

Cooking Time: 10 minutes

Servings: 6

Nutrition: Calories: 35 Fat: 0g Protein: 3g Carbohydrates: 7g Fiber: 4g Sugar: 4g Sodium: 236mg

Ingredients:

- 1 large head cauliflower
- 1 cup water
- ½ teaspoon salt
- 1 teaspoon red pepper flakes (optional)

Directions:

1. Remove any leaves from the cauliflower, and cut it into florets. In a large saucepan, bring the water to a boil.
2. Place a steamer basket over the water, and add the florets and salt. Cover and steam for 5 to 7 minutes, until tender.
3. In a large bowl, toss the cauliflower with the red pepper flakes (if using).
4. Transfer the florets to a large airtight container or 6 single-serving containers.
5. Let cool before sealing the lids.

58) Smoky Coleslaw

Preparation Time: 10 minutes

Cooking Time: 0 minute

Servings: 6

Nutrition: Calories: 73 Fat: 4g Protein: 1g Carbohydrates: 8g Fiber: 2g Sugar: 5g Sodium: 283mg

Ingredients:

- 1-pound shredded cabbage
- ⅓ cup vegan mayonnaise
- ¼ cup unseasoned rice vinegar
- 3 tablespoons plain vegan yogurt or plain soymilk
- 1 tablespoon vegan sugar
- ½ teaspoon salt
- ¼ teaspoon freshly ground black pepper
- ¼ teaspoon smoked paprika
- ¼ teaspoon chipotle powder

Directions:

1. Put the shredded cabbage in a large bowl.
2. In a medium bowl, whisk the mayonnaise, vinegar, yogurt, sugar, salt, pepper, paprika, and chipotle powder.
3. Pour over the cabbage, and mix with a spoon or spatula and until the cabbage shreds are coated.
4. Divide the coleslaw evenly among 6 single-serving containers.
5. Seal the lids.

59) Baked Potatoes

Preparation Time: 5 minutes

Cooking Time: 60 minutes

Servings: 5

Nutrition: Calories: 171 Fat: 3g Protein: 4g Carbohydrates: 34g Fiber: 5g Sugar: 3g Sodium: 129mg

Ingredients:

- 5 medium Russet potatoes or a variety of potatoes, washed and patted dry
- 1 to 2 tablespoons extra-virgin olive oil
- ¼ teaspoon salt
- ¼ teaspoon freshly ground black pepper

Directions:

1. Preheat the oven to 400°F. Pierce each potato several times with a fork or a knife.
2. Brush the olive oil over the potatoes, then rub each with a pinch of the salt and a pinch of the pepper.
3. Place the potatoes on a baking sheet and bake for 50 to 60 minutes, until tender.
4. Place the potatoes on a baking rack and cool completely.
5. Transfer to an airtight container or 5 single-serving containers.
6. Let cool before sealing the lids.

60) Asian Noodles

Preparation Time: 10 minutes

Cooking Time: 20 minutes

Servings: 4

Nutrition: Calories: 25; Fat: 2.0gProtein: 5.2g Carbohydrates: 5.3g Fiber: 4g;Sodium: 18mg

Ingredients:

- ½ cup peas
- 1 teaspoon rice vinegar
- 3 carrots, chopped
- 1 small packet vermicelli
- 3 tablespoons sesame oil
- 1 red pepper, chopped in small cubes
- 1 can baby corn
- 1 clove garlic, chopped
- 2 tablespoons soy sauce
- 1 teaspoon ginger powder
- ½ teaspoon curry powder
- Salt and black pepper, to taste

Directions:

1. Take a bowl and add ginger powder, vinegar, soy sauce, curry powder, and a pinch of salt to it.
2. Cook the noodles according to the instructions and drain them.
3. Heat the sesame oil and cook vegetables in it for 10 minutes on medium heat.
4. Add noodles to it and cook for 3 more minutes.
5. Remove from heat and serve to enjoy.

Plant Based Main Dishes Recipe

61) *Bean Burritos*

Preparation Time: 10 minutes

Cooking Time: 15 minutes

Servings: 8

Nutrition: Calories 290, Carbs 49 g, Fats 6 g, Protein 9 g

Ingredients:

- 32 oz. fat-free refried beans
- 6 tortillas
- 2 c. cooked rice
- ½ c. salsa
- 1 tbsp. olive oil
- 1 bunch green onions, chopped
- 2 bell peppers, chopped
- Guacamole

Directions:

1. Preheat the oven to 375°F.
2. Dump the refried beans into a saucepan and place over medium heat to warm.
3. Heat the tortillas and lay them out on a flat surface.
4. Spoon the beans in a long mound that runs across the tortilla, just a little off from center.
5. Spoon some rice and salsa over the beans; add the green pepper and onions to taste, along with any other finely chopped vegetables you like.
6. Fold over the shortest edge of the plain tortilla and roll it up, folding in the sides as you go.
7. Place each burrito, seam side down, on a nonstick-sprayed baking sheet.
8. Brush with olive oil and bake for 15 minutes.

62) *Chickpea Cutlets*

Preparation Time: 10 minutes

Cooking Time: 30 minutes

Servings: 12

Nutrition: Calories: 200, Protein: 8 g, Fat: 11g, Carbs: 21 g

Ingredients:

- 1 Red Bell Pepper
- 19 oz. Chickpeas, Rinsed & Drained
- 1 c. ground Almonds
- 2 tsps. Dijon Mustard
- 1 tsp. Oregano
- ½ tsp. Sage
- 1 c. Spinach, Fresh
- 1½ c. Rolled Oats
- 1 Clove Garlic, Pressed
- ½ Lemon, Juiced
- 2 tsps. Maple Syrup, Pure

Directions:

1. Get out a baking sheet. Line it with parchment paper.
2. Cut your red pepper in half and then take the seeds out. Place it on your baking sheet, and roast in the oven while you prepare your other ingredients.
3. Process your chickpeas, almonds, mustard, and maple syrup together in a food processor.
4. Add in your lemon juice, oregano, sage, garlic, and spinach, processing again. Make sure it's combined, but don't puree it.
5. Once your red bell pepper is softened, which should roughly take ten minutes, add this to the processor as well. Add in your oats, mixing well.
6. Form twelve patties, cooking in the oven for a half hour. They should be browned.

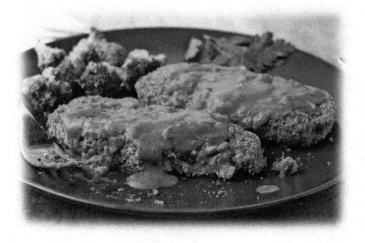

63) *Artichoke Sandwich*

Preparation time: 15 minutes

Cooking time: 10 minutes

Servings: 4

Nutrition: 220 Cal; 8 g Fat; 1 g Saturated Fat; 28 g Carbohydrates; 8 g Fiber; 2 g Sugars; 12 g Protein; 5g

Ingredients:

- 1 ¼ cooked white beans
- ½ cup cashew nuts
- 6 artichoke hearts, chopped
- ¼ cup sunflower seeds, hulled
- 1 clove of garlic, peeled
- ¼ teaspoon salt
- ¼ teaspoon ground black pepper
- 1 teaspoon dried rosemary
- 1 lemon, grated
- 6 tablespoons almond milk, unsweetened
- 8 pieces of rustic bread

Directions:

1. Soak cashew nuts in warm water for 10 minutes, then drain them and transfer into a food processor.
2. Add garlic, salt, black pepper, rosemary, lemon zest, and milk and then pulse for 2 minutes until smooth, scraping the sides of the container frequently.
3. Take a medium bowl, place beans in it, mash them by using a fork, then add sunflower seeds and artichokes and stir until mixed.
4. Pour in cashew nuts dressing, stir until coated, and taste to adjust seasoning.
5. Take a medium skillet pan, place it over medium heat, add bread slices, and cook for 3 minutes per side until toasted.
6. Spread white beans mixture on one side of four bread slices and then cover with the other four slices.
7. Serve straight away.

64) *Tofu Sandwich*

Preparation time: 10 minutes

Cooking time: 15 minutes

Servings: 4

Nutrition: 277 Cal;9.1 g Fat; 1.5 g Saturated Fat; 33.1 g Carbohydrates; 3.6 g Fiber; 12.7 g Sugars; 16.1 g Protein; 3g

Ingredients:

- 2 blocks of tofu, firm, pressed, drain
- 8 slices of tomato
- 8 leaves of lettuce
- 1 ½ teaspoon dried oregano
- ½ cup green pesto
- 2 tablespoons olive oil
- 8 slices of sandwich bread

Directions:

1. Switch on the oven, then set it to 375 degrees F and let it preheat.
2. Cut tofu into thick slices, place them in a baking sheet, drizzle with oil and sprinkle with oregano, and bake the tofu pieces for 15 minutes until roasted.
3. Assemble the sandwich and for this, spread pesto on one side of each bread slice, then top four slices with lettuce, tomato slices, and roasted tofu and then cover with the other four slices.
4. Serve straight away.

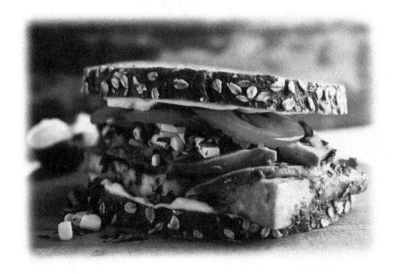

65) Taco Boats

Preparation time: 10 minutes

Cooking time: 0 minutes

Serving: 4

Nutrition: 314 Cal; 23.6 g Fat; 4 g Saturated Fat; 23.2 g Carbohydrates; 9.3 g Fiber; 6.2 g Sugars; 8 g Protein; 4g

Ingredients:

- 1 head romaine lettuce, destemmed
- For the Filling:
- 1/2 cup alfalfa sprouts
- 1 medium avocado, peeled, pitted, cubed
- 1 cup shredded carrots
- 1 cup halved cherry tomatoes
- 3/4 cup sliced red cabbage
- 1/2 cup sprouted hummus dip
- 1 tablespoon hemp seeds

For the Sauce:

- 1 tablespoon maple syrup
- 1/3 cup tahini
- 1/8 teaspoon sea salt
- 2 tablespoons lemon juice
- 3 tablespoons water

Directions:

1. Prepare the sauce and for this, take a medium bowl, add all the ingredients in it and whisk until well combined.
2. Assemble the boats and for this, arrange lettuce leaves in twelve portions, top each with hummus, and the remaining ingredients for the filling.
3. Serve with prepared sauce.

66) Veggie Tuna Salad

Preparation time: 10 minutes

Cooking time: 0 minutes

Serving: 4

Nutrition: 207 Cal;7 g Fat; 1 g Saturated Fat; 27 g Carbohydrates;8 g Fiber;1 g Sugars; 9 g Protein; 3g

Ingredients:

- 1/2 cup chopped celery
- 3 cups cooked chickpeas
- 1 tablespoon capers, chopped
- 2 tablespoons sweet pickle relish
- 1 tablespoon yellow mustard paste
- 2 tablespoons mayonnaise

Directions:

1. Take a medium bowl, place chickpeas in it, add mustard and mayonnaise and mash by using a fork until peas are broken.
2. Add remaining ingredients and stir until well combined.
3. Serve straight away.

67) The Hippie Bowl

Preparation time: 20 minutes

Cooking time: 30 minutes

Servings: 2

Ingredients:

- 1½ cups cooked grains or roasted potatoes
- 1 (15-ounce) can beans, drained and rinsed, or 1½ cups cooked beans
- 4 to 5 cups cooked or raw vegetables

Direction:

SPICY BOWL

1. Cooked brown rice
2. Pinto beans simmered in vegetable broth with ground cumin and chili powder
3. Steamed kale tossed with lime juice

CURRY BOWL

1. Roasted Yukon Gold potatoes
2. Chickpeas or lentils simmered in coconut milk with spinach, ground turmeric, curry powder, and ground ginger

LITTLE ITALY BOWL

1. Cooked farro
2. Cannellini beans and diced tomatoes simmered with arugula, capers, dried oregano, dried basil, and dried parsley
3. Spoon the cooked grains or roasted potatoes into bowls. Top with the cooked beans and veggies.

Nutrition: Calories: 594; Saturated Fat: 1g; Total Fat: 4g; Protein: 28g; Total Carbs: 113g; Fiber: 34g; Sodium: 137mg

68) Tofu Ribbs

Preparation time: 1 hour

Cooking time: 30 minutes

Servings: 10

Nutrition: Calories: 227; Saturated Fat: 1g; Total Fat: 6g; Protein: 12g; Total Carbs: 35g; Fiber: 2g; Sodium: 76mg

Ingredients:

- 1 (14-ounce) block extra-firm tofu, pressed and drained
- 1 (14-ounce) can jackfruit, drained
- 1 cup chopped mushrooms (any kind)
- ¼ cup nutritional yeast
- 2 tablespoons ground flaxseed
- ½ cup BBQ Sauce

Direction:

1. Preheat the oven to 375°F. Line an 8-inch square baking pan with parchment paper.
2. In a food processor, combine the tofu, jackfruit, and mushrooms and pulse to chop and form a chunky texture.
3. Transfer the mixture to a medium bowl. Add the nutritional yeast and ground flaxseed and stir to combine.
4. Spread ¼ cup of BBQ sauce over the bottom of the prepared baking pan. Transfer the tofu mixture to the pan and spread it out evenly with a spatula.
5. Pour the remaining ¼ cup of BBQ sauce over the top and spread it evenly to cover the tofu mixture.
6. Bake for 30 minutes. Transfer the pan to a wire rack and let cool for 30 minutes.
7. Cut into 10 "ribs" and serve.

69) Spaghetti Marinara

Preparation time: 20 minutes

Cooking time: 30 minutes

Servings: 6

Nutrition: Calories: 102; Saturated Fat: 0g; Total Fat: 3g; Protein: 5g; Total Carbs: 16g; Fiber: 5g; Sodium: 178mg

Ingredients:

- 2 tablespoons Vegetable Broth
- 1 teaspoon minced garlic
- 4 medium zucchini, spiralized
- ½ teaspoon dried basil
- ½ teaspoon dried oregano
- ¼ to ½ teaspoon red pepper flakes
- ¼ teaspoon salt (optional)
- ¼ teaspoon freshly ground black pepper
- 2 cups "Meaty" Marinara

Direction:

1. In a large skillet, heat the broth over medium-high heat.
2. Add the garlic, zucchini, basil, oregano, red pepper flakes, salt (if using), and black pepper and sauté until the zucchini is barely tender, 1 to 2 minutes.
3. Divide the zoodles evenly among four bowls.
4. Spoon ½ cup of hot marinara sauce over each bowl and serve.

70) Quinoa Pilaf

Preparation time: 20 minutes

Cooking time: 30 minutes

Servings: 6

Nutrition: Calories: 230; Saturated Fat: 1g; Total Fat: 7g; Protein: 8g; Total Carbs: 34g; Fiber: 5g; Sodium: 37mg

Ingredients:

- ½ cup chopped red onion
- 1 cup diced carrots
- ½ teaspoon dried parsley
- ½ teaspoon dried thyme
- 1 cup dry quinoa, rinsed and drained
- 1½ cups Vegetable Broth
- ¼ cup chopped walnuts
- Chopped fresh parsley or thyme, for garnish

Direction:

1. In a large saucepan, dry sauté the onion and carrots over medium-high heat, stirring frequently to prevent sticking, until the onion is tender, 3 to 5 minutes.
2. Add the parsley, thyme, quinoa, and broth and bring to a boil.
3. Lower the heat to medium-low, cover, and cook for 15 minutes.
4. Remove the pan from the heat and let sit for 5 minutes.
5. Fluff the quinoa with a fork, add the walnuts, and gently mix until combined.
6. Spoon into bowls and serve garnished with fresh parsley.

71) Cheese Roulades

Preparation Time: 20 minutes

Cooking Time: 10 minutes

Servings: 24

Nutrition: Calories 24Carbohydrates 2g Fiber 0g Sugar 1g Cholesterol 4mg Total Fat 1g Protein 2g

Ingredients:

- 4 zucchini
- 2 tablespoons basil, minced
- 1 tablespoon Greek olives, chopped
- 1 teaspoon lemon zest, grated
- 1 tablespoon drained capers
- ¼ cup Parmesan cheese, grated
- 1 cup ricotta cheese
- 1/8 teaspoon pepper
- 1/8 teaspoon salt

Directions:

1. Mix everything except the zucchini in a bowl.
2. Slice the zucchini lengthwise into 24, 1-inch pieces.
3. Cook the zucchini pieces in batches in your greased grill rack over medium heat.
4. Grill each side for 2 to 3 minutes. They should be tender.
5. Keep the ricotta mix at the side of the zucchini slices.
6. Roll them up. Secure with toothpicks.

72) Oatmeal Butterscotch Cookies

Preparation Time: 10 minutes

Cooking Time: 15 minutes

Serves: 4 dozen

Nutrition: Calories 130 Carbohydrates 16g Cholesterol 20mg Fat 7g Protein 1g Sodium 90mg

Ingredients:

- ½ teaspoon cinnamon, ground
- 3 cups oats
- 2 eggs
- 1 teaspoon of baking soda
- 1-1/4 all-purpose flour
- 1 cup margarine or butter
- 1 teaspoon vanilla extract
- ½ teaspoon salt

Directions:

1. Preheat your oven to 350 °F.
2. Bring together the baking soda, flour, salt and cinnamon in a bowl.
3. Beat the eggs, vanilla extract and butter in a mixer bowl.
4. Beat in the flour mix gradually.
5. Stir in the oats.
6. Place rounded tablespoons on baking sheets. Bake for 5-6 minutes.
7. Let it cool for a couple of minutes.

73) Speedy Italian Balls

Preparation Time: 5 minutes

Cooking Time: 0 minutes

Servings: 2

Nutrition: Calories 175 Fat: 13.7g Net Carbs: 1.1g Protein: 11g

Ingredients:

- 2 oz bresaola, chopped
- 2 oz ricotta cheese, crumbled
- 2 tbsp mayonnaise
- 6 green olives, pitted and chopped
- ½ tbsp fresh basil, finely chopped

Directions:

1. In a bowl, mix mayonnaise, bresaola and ricotta cheese.
2. Place in fresh basil and green olives.
3. Form balls from the mixture and refrigerate.
4. Serve chilled.

74) Hard Boiled Eggs Stuffed

Preparation Time: 15 minutes

Cooking Time: 15 minutes

Servings: 2

Nutrition: Calories 173 Fat: 12.5g Net Carbs: 1.5g Protein: 13.6g

Ingredients:

- 4 eggs
- 1 tbsp green tabasco
- 2 tbsp Greek yogurt
- 2 tbsp ricotta cheese
- Salt to taste

Directions:

1. Cover the eggs with salted water and bring to a boil over medium heat for 10 minutes.
2. Place the eggs in an ice bath and let cool for 10 minutes.
3. Peel and slice in half lengthwise. Scoop out the yolks to a bowl; mash with a fork.
4. Whisk together the tabasco, Greek yogurt, ricotta cheese, mashed yolks, and salt, in a bowl.
5. Spoon this mixture into egg white.
6. Arrange on a serving plate to serve.

75) Coco-Macadamia Bombs

Preparation Time: 5 minutes

Cooking Time: 0 minutes

Servings: 16

Nutrition: 255 calories 25.5g fat 3.5g protein 7g carbs 3g fiber 4g net carbs

Ingredients:

- 1 cup coconut oil
- 1 cup smooth almond butter
- ½ cup unsweetened cocoa powder
- ¼ cup coconut flour
- Liquid stevia extract, to taste
- 16 whole macadamia nuts, raw

Directions:

- Melt the coconut oil and cashew butter together in a small saucepan.
- Whisk in the cocoa powder, coconut flour, and liquid stevia to taste.
- Remove from heat and let cool until it hardens slightly.
- Divide the mixture into 16 even pieces.
- Roll each piece into a ball around a macadamia nut and chill until ready to eat.

76) Almond Fat Bombs

Preparation Time: 5 minutes

Cooking Time: 0 minutes

Servings: 16

Nutrition: 260 calories 26g fat 4g protein 6g carbs 2g fiber 4g net

Ingredients:

- 1 cup coconut oil
- 1 cup smooth almond butter
- ½ cup unsweetened cocoa powder
- ¼ cup almond flour
- Liquid stevia extract, to taste
- ½ cup toasted sesame seeds

Directions:

1. Combine the coconut oil and almond butter in a small saucepan.
2. Cook over low heat until melted, then whisk in the cocoa powder, almond flour, and liquid stevia.
3. Remove from heat and let cool until it hardens slightly.
4. Divide the mixture into 16 even pieces and roll into balls. Roll the balls in the toasted sesame seeds and chill until ready to eat.

77) Tomato Gazpacho

Preparation Time: 2 hours and 25 minutes

Cooking Time: 0 minutes

Servings: 6

Nutrition: Calories: 181 Protein: 3 Grams Fat: 14 Grams Carbs: 14 Grams

Ingredients:

- 2 Tablespoons + 1 Teaspoon Red Wine Vinegar, Divided
- ½ Teaspoon Pepper
- 1 Teaspoon Sea Salt
- 1 Avocado,
- ¼ Cup Basil, Fresh & Chopped
- 3 Tablespoons + 2 Teaspoons Olive Oil, Divided
- 1 Clove Garlic, crushed
- 1 Red Bell Pepper, Sliced & Seeded
- 1 Cucumber, Chunked
- 2 ½ lbs. Large Tomatoes, Cored & Chopped

Directions:

1. Place half of your cucumber, bell pepper, and ¼ cup of each tomato in a bowl, covering. Set it in the fried.
2. Puree your remaining tomatoes, cucumber and bell pepper with garlic, three tablespoons oil, two tablespoons of vinegar, sea salt and black pepper into a blender, blending until smooth. Transfer it to a bowl, and chill for two hours.
3. Chop the avocado, adding it to your chopped vegetables, adding your remaining oil, vinegar, salt, pepper and basil.
4. Ladle your tomato puree mixture into bowls, and serve with chopped vegetables as a salad.

78) Italian Green salad

Preparation Time: 10 minutes

Cooking Time: 5 minutes

Servings: 4

Nutrition: Calories: 242; Total fat: 9g; Total carbs: 35g; Fiber: 10g; Sugar: 8g; Protein: 9g; Sodium: 688mg

Ingredients:

- one head of green lettuce, washed and drained
- 1 cucumber, sliced
- a bunch of radishes, sliced
- a bunch of spring onions, finely cut
- the juice of half a lemon or 2 tbsp of white wine vinegar
- 3 tbsp sunflower or olive oil
- salt, to taste

Directions:

1. Cut the lettuce into thin strips. Slice the cucumber and the radishes as thinly as possible and chop the spring onions.
2. Mix all the salad ingredients in a large salad bowl; add the lemon juice and oil and season with salt to taste.

79) *Russian salad*

Preparation Time: 15 minutes

Cooking Time: 5 minutes

Servings: 4

Nutrition: Calories: 326; Total fat: 24g; Total carbs: 22g; Fiber: 4g; Sugar: 7g; Protein: 8g; Sodium: 573mg

Ingredients:

- 3 potatoes
- 2 carrots
- 1 cup green peas, cooked, drained
- 1 cup mayonnaise
- 5-6 pickled gherkins, chopped
- salt, to taste
- 6-7 black olives, to serve

Directions:

1. Boil the potatoes and carrots, then chop into small cubes.
2. Put everything, except for the mayonnaise, in a serving bowl and mix.
3. Add salt to taste, then stir in the mayonnaise.
4. Garnish with parsley and olives.
5. Serve cold.

80) *Italian Potato Salad*

Preparation Time: 10 minutes

Cooking Time: 5 minutes

Servings: 4

Nutrition: Calories: 238; Total fat: 1g;Total carbs: 46g; Fiber: 7g; Sugar: 29g; Protein: 16g; Sodium: 15mg

Ingredients:

- 4-5 large potatoes
- 2-3 spring onions, finely chopped
- juice of ½ a lemon
- 5 tbsp sunflower or olive oil
- salt and pepper, to taste
- fresh parsley

Directions:

1. Peel and boil the potatoes for about 20-25 minutes, drain and leave to cool.
2. In a salad bowl add the finely chopped spring onions, the lemon juice, salt, pepper and olive oil, and mix gently.
3. Cut the potatoes into cubes and add to the salad bowl.
4. Gently mix, sprinkle with parsley.
5. Serve cold.

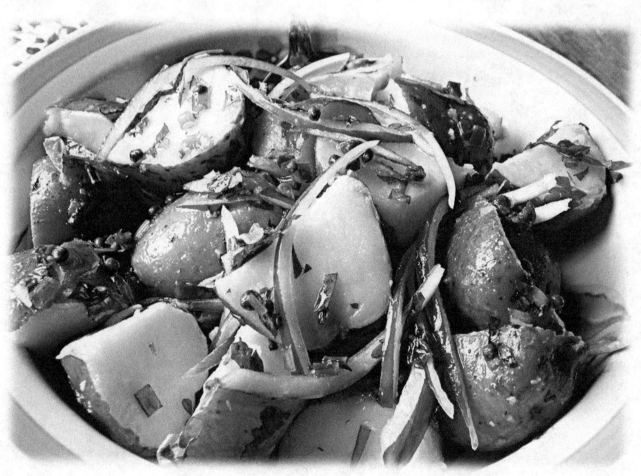

Plant Based Drinks & Smoothies

81) Hazelnut and Chocolate Milk

Preparation time: 5 minutes

Cooking time: 0 minute

Servings: 2

Nutrition: Calories: 120 Cal Fat: 5 g Carbs: 19 g Protein: 2 g Fiber: 1 g

Ingredients:
- 2 tablespoons cocoa powder
- 4 dates, pitted
- 1 cup hazelnuts
- 3 cups of water

Direction:
1. Place all the ingredients in the order in a food processor or blender and then pulse for 2 to 3 minutes at high speed until smooth.
2. Pour the smoothie into two glasses and then serve.

82) Sweet and Sour Juice

Preparation time: 5 minutes

Cooking time: 0 minute

Servings: 2

Nutrition: Calories: 90 Cal Fat: 0 g Carbs: 23 g Protein: 0 g Fiber: 9 g

Ingredients:
- 2 medium apples, cored, peeled, chopped
- 2 large cucumbers, peeled
- 4 cups chopped grapefruit
- 1 cup mint

Directions:
1. Process all the ingredients in the order in a juicer or blender and then strain it into two glasses.
2. Serve straight away.

83) Chocolate and Cherry Smoothie

Preparation time: 5 minutes

Cooking time: 0 minute

Servings: 2

Nutrition: Calories: 324 Cal Fat: 5 g Carbs: 75.1 g Protein: 7.2 g Fiber: 11.3 g

Ingredients:
- 4 cups frozen cherries
- 2 tablespoons cocoa powder
- 1 scoop of protein powder
- 1 teaspoon maple syrup
- 2 cups almond milk, unsweetened

Directions:
1. Place all the ingredients in the order in a food processor or blender and then pulse for 2 to 3 minutes at high speed until smooth.
2. Pour the smoothie into two glasses and then serve.

84) Berry Lemonade tea

Preparation Time: 5 minutes

Cooking Time: 12 minutes

Servings: 4

Nutrition: Calories 21; Carbs 8g; Fat 0.2g; Protein 0.4g

Ingredients:
- 3 tea bags
- 2 cups of natural lemonade
- 1 cup of frozen mixed berries
- 2 cups of water
- 1 lemon, sliced

Directions:
1. Put everything in the Instant Pot and cover. Cook on High for 12 minutes.
2. Open, strain, and serve.

85) Swedish Glögg

Preparation Time: 5 minutes

Cooking Time: 15 minutes

Servings: 1

Nutrition: Calories 194;Carbs 41g; Fat 3g; Protein 1.7g

Ingredients:
- ½ cup of orange juice
- ½ cup of water
- 1 piece of ginger cut into ½ pieces
- 1 whole clove
- 1 opened cardamom pods
- 2 tbsps. orange zest
- 1 cinnamon stick
- 1 whole allspice
- 1 vanilla bean

Directions:
1. Add everything in the pot.
2. Cover and cook on High for 15 minutes.
3. Open and serve.

86) Spiced Ginger Cider

Preparation Time: 5 minutes

Cooking Time: 13 minutes

Servings: 12

Nutrition: Calories 141; Carbs 35.2g; Fat 0.6g; Protein 0.4g

Ingredients:

- 2 small apples, peeled
- 12 cups apple cider
- 2 whole allspice
- 2 tsps. fresh ginger
- 4 tsps. orange zest
- 2 tsps. cinnamon powder
- 4 whole cloves
- ½ tsp. ground nutmeg

Directions:

1. Put everything in the pot.
2. Cover and cook on High for 13 minutes.
3. Open, strain, and serve.

87) Tasty Ranch Dressing/dip

Preparation Time: 5 minutes

Cooking Time: 10 minutes

Servings: 2

Nutrition: Calories: 100 Cal Fat: 2 g Carbs: 10 g Protein: 10 g Fiber: 10 g

Ingredients:

- ½ c. soy milk, unsweetened
- 1 tbsp. dill, chopped
- 2 t. parsley, chopped
- ¼ t. black pepper
- ½ t. of the following:
- onion powder
- garlic powder
- 1 c. vegan mayonnaise

Directions:

1. In a medium bowl, whisk all the ingredients together until smooth.
2. If dressing is too thick, add ¼ tablespoon of soy milk at a time until the desired consistency.
3. Transfer to an airtight container or jar and refrigerate for 1 hour.
4. Serve over leafy greens or as a dip.

88) Brownie Batter Orange Chia Shake

Preparation time: 5 minutes

Cooking time: 0 minute

Servings: 2

Nutrition: Calories: 487 Cal Fat: 31 g Carbs: 57 g Protein: 9 g Fiber: 11 g

Ingredients:

- 2 tablespoons cocoa powder
- 3 tablespoons chia seeds
- ¼ teaspoon salt
- 4 tablespoons chocolate chips
- 4 teaspoons coconut sugar
- ½ teaspoon orange zest
- ½ teaspoon vanilla extract, unsweetened
- 2 cup almond milk

Directions:

1. Place all the ingredients in the order in a food processor or blender and then pulse for 2 to 3 minutes at high speed until smooth.
2. Pour the smoothie into two glasses and then serve

89) Pumpkin Spice Frappuccino

Preparation time: 5 minutes

Cooking time: 0 minute

Servings: 2

Nutrition: Calories: 90 Cal Fat: 6 g Carbs: 5 g Protein: 2 g Fiber: 1 g

Ingredients:

- ½ teaspoon ground ginger
- 1/8 teaspoon allspice
- ½ teaspoon ground cinnamon
- 2 tablespoons coconut sugar
- 1/8 teaspoon nutmeg
- ¼ teaspoon ground cloves
- 1 teaspoon vanilla extract, unsweetened
- 2 teaspoons instant coffee
- 2 cups almond milk, unsweetened
- 1 cup of ice cubes

Directions:

1. Place all the ingredients in the order in a food processor or blender and then pulse for 2 to 3 minutes at high speed until smooth.
2. Pour the Frappuccino into two glasses and then serve.

90) Blueberry, Hazelnut and Hemp Smoothie

Preparation time: 5 minutes

Cooking time: 0 minute

Servings: 2

Nutrition: Calories: 376 Cal Fat: 25 g Carbs: 26 g Protein: 14 g Fiber: 4 g

Ingredients:

- 2 tablespoons hemp seeds
- 1 ½ cups frozen blueberries
- 2 tablespoons chocolate protein powder
- 1/2 teaspoon vanilla extract, unsweetened
- 2 tablespoons chocolate hazelnut butter
- 1 small frozen banana
- 3/4 cup almond milk

Directions:

1. Place all the ingredients in the order in a food processor or blender and then pulse for 2 to 3 minutes at high speed until smooth.
2. Pour the smoothie into two glasses and then serve.

91) Berry and Yogurt Smoothie

Preparation time: 5 minutes

Cooking time: 0 minute

Servings: 2

Nutrition: Calories: 326 Cal Fat: 6.5 g Carbs: 65.6 g Protein: 8 g Fiber: 8.4 g

Ingredients:

- 2 small bananas
- 3 cups frozen mixed berries
- 1 ½ cup cashew yogurt
- 1/2 teaspoon vanilla extract, unsweetened
- 1/2 cup almond milk, unsweetened

Directions:

1. Place all the ingredients in the order in a food processor or blender and then pulse for 2 to 3 minutes at high speed until smooth.
2. Pour the smoothie into two glasses and then serve.

92) Strawberry and Chocolate Milkshake

Preparation time: 5 minutes

Cooking time: 0 minute

Servings: 2

Nutrition: Calories: 199 Cal Fat: 4.1 g Carbs: 40.5 g Protein: 3.7 g Fiber: 5.5 g

Ingredients:

- 2 cups frozen strawberries
- 3 tablespoons cocoa powder
- 1 scoop protein powder
- 2 tablespoons maple syrup
- 1 teaspoon vanilla extract, unsweetened
- 2 cups almond milk, unsweetened

Directions:

1. Place all the ingredients in the order in a food processor or blender and then pulse for 2 to 3 minutes at high speed until smooth.
2. Pour the smoothie into two glasses and then serve.

93) 'Sweet Tang' and Chia Smoothie

Preparation time: 5 minutes

Cooking time: 0 minute

Servings: 2

Nutrition: Calories: 406 Cal Fat: 9.3 g Carbs: 77.4 g Protein: 6.3 g Fiber: 13 g

Ingredients:

- 4 large plums
- 2 tablespoon chia seeds
- 1/2 cup pineapple chunks
- 1/2 cup ice cubes
- 3/4 cup coconut water

Directions:

1. Place all the ingredients in the order in a food processor or blender and then pulse for 2 to 3 minutes at high speed until smooth.
2. Pour the smoothie into two glasses and then serve.

94) Strawberry, Blueberry and Banana Smoothie

Preparation time: 5 minutes

Cooking time: 0 minute

Servings: 2

Nutrition: Calories: 334 Cal Fat: 17 g Carbs: 46 g Protein: 7 g Fiber: 7 g

Ingredients:

- 1 tablespoon hulled hemp seeds
- ½ cup of frozen strawberries
- 1 small frozen banana
- ½ cup frozen blueberries
- 2 tablespoons cashew butter
- ¾ cup cashew milk, unsweetened

Directions:

1. Place all the ingredients in the order in a food processor or blender and then pulse for 2 to 3 minutes at high speed until smooth.
2. Pour the smoothie into two glasses and then serve.

95) Green Lemonade

Preparation time: 5 minutes

Cooking time: 0 minute

Servings: 2

Nutrition: Calories: 102.3 Cal Fat: 1.1 g Carbs: 26.2 g Protein: 4.7 g Fiber: 8.5 g

Ingredients:

- 10 large stalks of celery, chopped
- 2 medium green apples, cored, peeled, chopped
- 2 medium cucumbers, peeled, chopped
- 2 inches piece of ginger
- 10 stalks of kale, chopped
- 2 cups parsley

Directions:

1. Process all the ingredients in the order in a juicer or blender and then strain it into two glasses.
2. Serve straight away.

96) Spiced Buttermilk

Preparation time: 5 minutes

Cooking time: 0 minute

Servings: 2

Nutrition: Calories: 92 Cal Fat: 2 g Carbs: 5 g Protein: 11 g Fiber: 0.5 g

Ingredients:

- 3/4 teaspoon ground cumin
- 1/4 teaspoon sea salt
- 1/8 teaspoon ground black pepper
- 2 mint leaves
- 1/8 teaspoon lemon juice
- ¼ cup cilantro leaves
- 1 cup of chilled water
- 1 cup vegan yogurt, unsweetened
- Ice as needed

Directions:

1. Place all the ingredients in the order in a food processor or blender, except for cilantro and ¼ teaspoon cumin, and then pulse for 2 to 3 minutes at high speed until smooth.
2. Pour the milk into glasses, top with cilantro and cumin, and then serve.

97) Mexican Hot Chocolate Mix

Preparation time: 5 minutes

Cooking time: 0 minute

Servings: 2

Nutrition: Calories: 127 Cal Fat: 5 g Carbs: 20 g Protein: 1 g Fiber: 2 g

Ingredients:

- 1/3 cup chopped dark chocolate
- 1/8 teaspoon cayenne
- 1/8 teaspoon salt
- 1/2 teaspoon cinnamon
- 1/4 cup coconut sugar
- 1 teaspoon cornstarch
- 3 tablespoons cocoa powder
- 1/2 teaspoon vanilla extract, unsweetened
- 2 cups milk, warmed

Directions:

1. Place all the ingredients of hot chocolate mix in the order in a food processor or blender and then pulse for 2 to 3 minutes at high speed until ground.
2. Stir 2 tablespoons of the chocolate mix into a glass of milk until combined and then serve.

98) Mocha Chocolate Shake

Preparation time: 5 minutes

Cooking time: 0 minute

Servings: 2

Nutrition: Calories: 357 Cal Fat: 21 g Carbs: 31 g Protein: 12 g Fiber: 5 g

Ingredients:

- 1/4 cup hemp seeds
- 2 teaspoons cocoa powder, unsweetened
- 1/2 cup dates, pitted
- 1 tablespoon instant coffee powder
- 2 tablespoons flax seeds
- 2 1/2 cups almond milk, unsweetened
- 1/2 cup crushed ice

Directions:

1. Place all the ingredients in the order in a food processor or blender and then pulse for 2 to 3 minutes at high speed until smooth.
2. Pour the smoothie into two glasses and then serve.

99) Red Beet, Pear and Apple Smoothie

Preparation time: 5 minutes

Cooking time: 0 minute

Servings: 2

Nutrition: Calories: 132 Cal Fat: 0 g Carbs: 34 g Protein: 1 g Fiber: 5 g

Ingredients:

- 1/2 of medium beet, peeled, chopped
- 1 tablespoon chopped cilantro
- 1 orange, juiced
- 1 medium pear, chopped
- 1 medium apple, cored, chopped
- 1/4 teaspoon ground black pepper
- 1/8 teaspoon rock salt
- 1 teaspoon coconut sugar
- 1/4 teaspoons salt
- 1 cup of water

Directions:

1. Place all the ingredients in the order in a food processor or blender and then pulse for 2 to 3 minutes at high speed until smooth.
2. Pour the smoothie into two glasses and then serve.

100) Banana and Protein Smoothie

Preparation time: 5 minutes

Cooking time: 0 minute

Servings: 2

Nutrition: Calories: 272 Cal Fat: 3.8 g Carbs: 59.4 g Protein: 4.3 g Fiber: 7.1 g

Ingredients:

- 2/3 cup frozen pineapple chunk
- 10 frozen strawberries
- 2 frozen bananas
- 2 scoops protein powder
- 2 teaspoons cocoa powder
- 2 tablespoons maple syrup
- 2 teaspoons vanilla extract, unsweetened
- 2 cups almond milk, unsweetened

Directions:

1. Place all the ingredients in the order in a food processor or blender and then pulse for 2 to 3 minutes at high speed until smooth.
2. Pour the smoothie into two glasses and then serve.

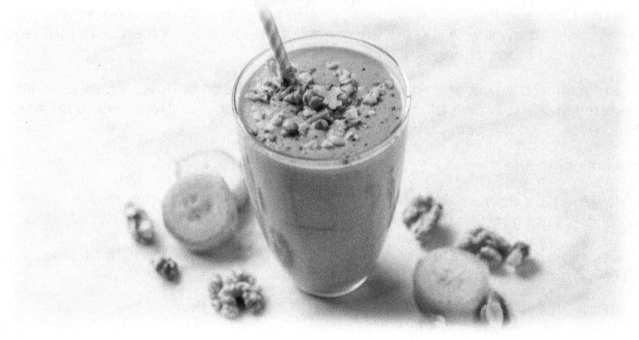

7. "The Smith's Meal Plan Protocol" – Women Version

The meal plan is divided into 7 days, to be repeated for 3 weeks, with 5 meals a day. At the end of the 21 days, the week is reversed as follows:

Day 1 = Day 7

Day 2 = Day 6

Day 3 = Day 5

Day 4 = Day 4

Day 5 = Day 3

Day 6 = Day 2

Day 7 = Day 1

And so on for another 3 weeks.

Following this plan does not guarantee extreme results.

The aim is to keep metabolism under control in order to change eating habits, have more energy available during the day, and keep under control the values that lead to hormonal sudden changes.

The plan here below is an example of food plan that can be followed by a healthy person without specific pathologies. I do not take responsibility for personal injury, before following the plan consult your doctor

Instructions for use

Follow the plan daily: drink plenty of water at every meal, it is imperative not to take alcohol (it's not good for the body!)

It is possible to substitute meals at will according to this book, so that it does not become habitual to always eat the same things.

Day 1

Pine Apple Smoothie | Calories 566 - **Page 11**

Plant Based Low Carb | Calories 40 - **Page 22**

Artichoke Sandwich | Calories 220 - **Page 40**

Potato and Carrots Salad | Calories 106 **Page 32**

Strawberry and Chocolate Milkshake | Calories 199 **Page 49**

Total Calories - 1131

Day 2

Choco Smoothies | Calories 474 **Page 11**

Veggie Chow | Calories 30 **Page 22**

Speedy Italian Balls | Calories 175 **Page 43**

Avocado Salad | Calories 224 **Page 32**

Spiced Ginger Cider | Calories 141 **Page 48**

Total Calories 1044

Day 3

Mixed Bowl | Calories 533 **Page 14**

Kale Chips | Calories 24 **Page 26**

Italian Green salad | Calories 242 **Page 44**

Stuffed Cauliflower | Calories 35 **Page 35**

Spiced Butter Milk | Calories 92 **Page 50**

Total Calories 926

Day 4

Berries with Muslie | Calories 441 **Page 12**

Chickpea with Cocco | Calories 225 **Page 24**

Russian Salad | Calories 326 **Page 45**

Pepper Salad | Calories 116 **Page 33**

Swedish Glögg | Calories 194 **Page 47**

Total Calories 1302

Day 5

A cup of Quinoa | Calories 392 **Page 12**

Tomatoes Mix and Basil | Calories 242 **Page 27**

The Hippie Bowl | Calories 594 **Page 41**

Veggie Rice Bowl | Calories 260 **Page 34**

Sweet and Sour Juice | Calories 120 **Page 47**

Total Calories 1608

Day 6

Oatmeal Pumk | Calories 218 **Page 13**

Pamplona Rice | Calories 242 **Page 28**

Bean Burritos | Calories 290 **Page 39**

Coconut Balls | Calories 88 **Page 32**

Pumpkin Spice Frappuccino | Calories 90 **Page 48**

Total Calories 928

Day 7

Sfilatino Banana Bread | Calories 178 **Page 13**

Sweet Potato with Black Bean | Calories 387 **Page 23**

Italian Potato Salad | Calories 238 **Page 45**

Grilled Asparagus with Chickpea | Calories 270 **Page 35**

Spiced Buttermilk | Calories 92 **Page 50**

Total Calories 1165